YOUR REAL BMI

Your Real BMI

a Better Me Index with Breath, Movement and Intake

CYNTHIA SCHAEFER

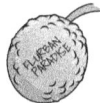

Flurban Paradise

Your Real BMI: A Better Me Index through Breath Movement and
Intake
by Cynthia Schaefer https://www.flurbanparadise.com
YouTube: https://bit.ly/Flurban
Find me on Amazon: https://amzn.to/434aRxp
Insta: https://www.instagram.com/flurban_paradise/
FB: https://www.facebook.com/Flurbanparadise

This book is dedicated to all of us who have struggled with finding a
way to be healthy and whole.

Publisher: Flurban Paradise
        4786 SW 72nd Ave.
        Davie, Florida 33314
        www.flurbanparadise.com

First Printing 2023

ISBN: 979-8-9893916-0-8

Special thanks to my editor, reviewers, and to all who have inspired
me:
Lily Abello [http://www.linkedin.com/in/lily-abello]

Contents

Medical Disclaimer

This book is intended for informational purposes only and does not serve as a replacement for professional medical advice, diagnosis, or treatment. The author and publisher are not medical professionals; the information presented herein is based on traditional knowledge, personal experiences, and research.

Always consult with a qualified healthcare provider or herbalist before making any changes to your diet, medications, or health routines, especially when introducing new herbs or supplements. Some herbs can interact with medications or have side effects. Every individual's body is unique, and what works for one person may not work for another.

Never disregard professional medical advice or delay seeking it because of something you have read in this book. If you think you may have a medical emergency, call your doctor, go to the emergency department, or call emergency services immediately.

The author and publisher disclaim any liability or loss, personal or otherwise, resulting from the procedures and information presented in this book.

Foreward

Can you imagine waking up every morning feeling great about your life, health, the day ahead, and all the days ahead? What would it feel like to wake with a clear head, naturally, and feel vitally alive from the moment you came awake until you fell into a deep, restorative sleep at the end of a day that you felt great about? This can be your life.

We all know how much sicker we are as a general population than we were 100 years ago. The correlation between technology and industrialism's rise to the increase in chronic disease and mental illness is apparent. What isn't clear to many is the solution.

Everyone wants to be healthy. The billions of dollars spent annually on supplements, books, gym memberships, and wellness coaches speak volumes about our society.

I want to share with you why I wrote this book and how I want to help you so that you don't have the struggles that I did.

I started to fall apart in my late twenties and early thirties. For me, it manifested mostly as depression and severe hormonal disruptions. I won't take you through the tale of woe, but I will tell you that the journey was long, painful, and could have been avoided if I'd had some basic understanding of the principles in this book.

The things that I learned along the way are the things that I'm sharing with you. I don't want you to take thirty years to find your bliss. I want you to find your bliss now, wherever you are in your life or however old or young you are. You can have a much better tomorrow if you follow the principles of this book.

It's simple, but it's not unless you know certain things. This book will give you the key to a lifetime of vibrant wellness.

Chapter 1

What We Really Need

I was in my early thirties, sitting at the doctor's office again. It was one of those practices with multiple doctors, and I was sitting with a doctor I hadn't met before. He was probably about my age, and I remember him as sweaty. He was also overweight, and his skin was pasty.

He slumped on the stool, not looking at me, as he scanned my file.

One of the odd things that I was experiencing had to do with my water consumption. If I didn't drink at least a gallon of water daily, I would experience symptoms like a urinary tract infection. I didn't have a UTI, or at least the test didn't show anything, but the pain, burning, and other symptoms remained.

The excess need for water (this was the early nineties before hydration was a thing) seemed to me to be a sign that something wasn't working right in my body.

The response from the doctor was deeply humiliating. I had been honest about my past, including past abuses of drugs and alcohol. When I asked him about my intense thirst and need for water (the test for diabetes was negative), he looked up sharply and, in a very loud voice, said, "You can't expect to do all those drugs and not have problems."

If only I had understood the importance of the message from my body. It was clearly telling me that my water element was out of balance.

I don't remember much more about the visit except walking out of the office and realizing as I passed another door and listened to the voices behind it that probably everyone in the office and waiting room had heard his condemnation of me.

During my next desperate visit to that office, they ran some tests that revealed that my thyroid was not producing adequately, and the medication they gave me helped for a short time. It was a step up from the total dismissal that I had gotten at the previous visit.

Each step in my search for wellness showed me another piece of the puzzle. One of the last pieces was my understanding that the entire system was flawed and that the doctor who humiliated me was as much a victim of the system as I was.

It was clear that his health was wrecked. When you realize that the methods they use to educate medical professionals are eerily like those used to brainwash or torture people, you can understand why our medical system is under so much strain. But that's only part of the problem.

We are the other part of the problem. I was raised in the paradigm that professionals had the answers, and their conclusions were never questioned. Medical professionals are meant to be acute care providers. We have tried to turn them into chronic care providers. This doesn't work for any of us.

If we really want a workable healthcare system, we must have a healthy population and make medical care about acute illnesses rather than chronic ones. This is how we all win.

People are desperately seeking help and access to wellness. They aren't finding it in this complicated world of superfoods and supplements. Processed foods are made to addict and confuse us. Supplements, powders, and superfoods all claim to be the answer, but they aren't. Medical providers offer us medications that have serious side effects. We are lost, confused, and unhealthy. We can change all that.

The irony is that the solution should be clear. It's pretty basic. But the "treat the disease" instead of the personal model of medicine has left us feeling as if we don't have control over our wellness. We give our power to the person giving us the pill, and we aren't getting the results we need. It is nobody's and everybody's fault at the time.

Many doctors are as frustrated by the current state of health care as we are. They feel driven by the HMOs and insurance companies. The amount of time they spend with each patient is less and less. They spent years of their lives and made great sacrifices to become healers. They want to help us. We're just expecting the wrong things from them.

In my wellness practice, I've worked with all sorts of people. One of my clients is a doctor who sends me many referrals. When she came to me, she told me she was lucky if she could have a bowel movement once a week. Despite her vast knowledge of the human body, she struggled with such a fundamental bodily function.

Her training didn't include understanding her particular body type and what foods and activities could lead her to vibrant, good health. With a few tweaks to her understanding of food and environmental toxins, she was on her way to vibrant wellness. A few simple changes transformed her wellness and reverberated through some ancillary health issues she was experiencing.

Her energy came back, and she said she felt years younger. She was more able to help her patients and incorporated her new understanding into her practice.

Nature works miracles in the human body. Through classes, consults, and mentoring, I've seen hundreds of people make radical changes to their lives based on understanding how their specific body works and how they can partner with nature to achieve vibrant wellness.

Vibrant wellness is our birthright, and having it changes everything. I've seen people find emotional wellness after years of struggle simply by understanding basic wellness principles.

HOW?

I'm using an acronym that you are probably familiar with - BMI. Instead of Body Mass Index, this acronym is the key to moving into a Better Me Initiative by understanding how the tools of Breath, Movement, and Intake work for you.

We will overcome the two things that keep most people from vibrant health:

1. Not knowing exactly what they should do to get consistent, long-term results.
2. Not being able to implement the things that need to happen because of motivation struggles or other limitations that aren't addressed by the types of changes they are trying to make.

As we go through the book, I will give you the framework, tools, and a complete roadmap to get you through the marvelous changes that will happen.

I'm probably going to give you too much information in some places. I do that sometimes. The thing is, I don't know how much information you need to move forward. Feel free to skip the parts containing information you already know or are in a format you aren't interested in.

FUTURE YOU!

People who are vibrantly alive live differently. There is more joy, resilience, and satisfaction in their lives. They live longer, fuller lives and have better relationships. This can be you. Let me introduce you to Future You.

Future You! When I first started imagining my Future Me, I always saw her in full superwoman mode. I even pictured Future Me in the cape and boots. I don't have the cape or the boots, but the Future Me is beyond what I had imagined.

The things that I learned on my journey were deeply empowering, and that's what I'm sharing with you. The tools I will share have been the basis of wellness across multiple cultures and thousands of years.

By choosing this book, you are giving Future You an entirely different trajectory than the one you might be on now. Small changes now can make enormous differences later.

Please take a moment now to close your eyes and picture Future You. What do you look like? How do you feel? Look forward 5, 10, 15 years. Are you the person that you want to be? If not, then let's make a new picture of Future You.

It doesn't matter how unlikely you think the things you want for Future You are. I never imagined in my early thirties that I'd end up doing any of the things I do today. We're not looking to be specific. Let's evoke the feelings first.

What does it feel like to live the life that Future You wants? What is it like waking up to the day? How do you feel about your day when you put your head on the pillow?

Waking up used to be awful for me. I was groggy, anxious, and miserable. My day would start with the jarring sound of the alarm, setting the tone for a day full of reactivity and an overstimulated nervous system.

Now, I wake up naturally. My first thoughts are usually of gratitude for the life I'm living. I wait for the rooster to crow before I get out of bed, and I feel good from the moment I'm awake.

How does Future You want to start their day? How will they feel, and what might they be thinking? When you meet Future You, it gives you a GPS point to move towards. It gives you someone to be accountable to and keeps the rewards present.

If you are already comfortable with visualizations, then go ahead and do your thing. Don't skip this step if you aren't skilled at it yet.

Let's lay our heads down at the end of Future Day with Future You. Do you go to sleep easily, knowing you gave yourself a day fully lived? Does your body relax easily and naturally? Is your mind content with what you accomplished so it does not need to keep you up with worries and to-do lists?

Vibrant wellness is a gift you give yourself and your loved ones. Bring them into the picture now. How do they benefit from Future You having vibrant wellness? Did you inspire them also to become fully alive? Were you a better parent, partner, or friend because of your commitment to be the best Future You?

Also, whenever you think about Future You, I want you to see them in a classic superhero pose with their hands on their hips. Give them a cape and a theme song. Make them real. Make them powerful. Do this often.

Creating Future You:

Now that you've met Future You, I want to take a moment to discuss something that will have a massive impact on Future You: Epigenetics.

Epigenetics is a branch of biology that studies heritable changes in gene expression (active versus inactive genes) that do not involve changes to the underlying DNA sequence. In other words, it's about how genes are turned "on" or "off" rather than changes in the genes themselves.

What is important for you to understand about epigenetics is that you can turn on and off gene expression. Understanding this helps you see how we consciously create Future You to be what you desire them to be.

Expressed simply, this means you can turn on the genes that will result in a longer healthspan and turn off the genes that trigger the start of chronic or deadly diseases. It's a bit more complex than that, but the bottom line is that you have a lot more control over how Future You feels and lives than you might think.

This is really exciting!!

Think about this for a moment. Think about loved ones you've lost or things you or people you love didn't get to do because they weren't healthy enough. Now, think about how differently things could have turned out if the gene that had caused the loss or illness had been turned off before it expressed and stayed off. What would you give for that power?

How do you turn genes on and off? The methods you have the most control over are choices you can make about how you think, what you allow into your body, and how you treat your body. Interestingly, when you look at the ancient wisdom of many traditional medicine practices, they align with our current understanding of how our choices can tremendously impact our well-being.

After all, you wouldn't stop brushing your teeth and expect the dentist to make everything okay on your annual visit. Yet that is what we do in many of our daily lifestyle choices, and then we get bad news at the doctor's office.

We will turn to ancient wisdom here and give you a guaranteed framework that will work for you. You'll have the tools to know your own Secret Formula of movements, breathwork, foods, and thoughts that work for you.

The other place where many of us get stuck is motivation. I think a good part of that comes from trying things that didn't work for us or not being sure that the things we were changing were really going to work.

Knowing that you are doing what your uniqueness calls for and having the tools to figure out what you can do that has the best results for exactly where you are at this moment in time is a powerful motivator.

With the framework you'll learn, you'll know it is for you and works for you. That will make all the difference in your motivation. You'll also have some tools that are game-changers in helping you with motivation. You'll notice changes quickly and know you're on the right track. Future You will slowly emerge from within.

Chapter 2

An Intuitive Framework

Traditional medicines like Ayurveda (Traditional Medicine from India), TCM (Traditional Chinese Medicine), and Herbalism have worked within frameworks that make diagnosing and treating minor imbalances easy to learn and understand. They knew it was far better to help people stay healthy than to try to fix things after the imbalances had gotten too far.

The framework that you will learn in this book is the foundation of all the ancient practices above. It will give you the ability to manage your wellness and create a new, healthier relationship between you and your body. It's the key to finding your Secret Formula.

Let's start by acknowledging that there are some things beyond our control. We live in a toxic world. We can't avoid some toxins, but many that we can.

Environmental toxins wreak havoc on our bodies, so avoiding them as much as possible is critical. EWG.org is a great resource for more knowledge about this. Spend time on the site, checking your cleaning and personal products and learning to avoid environmental toxins. If you want to dive deeper, there are a lot of great books on environmental toxins. DON'T SKIP THIS STEP!

Toxins can create cellular dysfunction, which will make everything harder. They will mess with your endocrine system, which will affect your metabolism. If you have weight that won't come off no matter what you do or problems that seem connected to hormonal imbalances, toxins probably play a part.

Let's say you wanted to get the house ready for a party. You know who you want to invite. You've got the food, the drinks, and the decorations figured out. The music playlist is ready.

What's the one thing everybody does before they throw a party? They clean the house. We don't put the decorations up over the cobwebs (unless it's Halloween!), The same principles apply to your body.

Make sure you aren't adding toxins. Remember that every new thing you buy has VOCs (volatile organic compounds) that you may inhale. What you can't avoid, you mitigate. This can be as simple as a HEPA filter in your house.

Toxins are a topic onto themselves. I follow these simple rules:

1. Anything that isn't essential oils but is scented is a hard no for me. Perfumes, body sprays, laundry detergents, air fresheners, scented toilet paper. Unless they have a green rating from EWG.org, they are probably disrupting your hormones.
2. I don't buy new if I can buy used. If I buy new, I find the least toxic choice, and then I run a HEPA filter near it until I think it's done off-gassing.

The good news is that many toxins will clear naturally from a healthy body. Awareness and avoiding the most obvious sources empower your body to eliminate accumulated toxins and repair itself naturally.

We control what we can, and don't dwell on what we can't.

Putting aside what we can't control, we can control a vast amount. We have the power to change so much.

The most important thing I want you to know right now is this: Your vibrant health blueprint is uniquely yours. That's why the things that might have worked for your sibling/co-worker/friend might not work for you.

More importantly, the single metric that most people use to determine if the changes they've made are working (How does my body look to others?) has little validity in how you're really doing.

That's why I used BMI as the acronym for your Secret Formula. The old BMI stood for Body Mass Index, a metric used to determine "appropriate" weight for individuals based on gender and height.

Instead of a disempowering metric focused on weight, you'll have a deeply empowering metric that considers all aspects of your thrivival.

Thrivival is my word for moving beyond survival and into a world where you are thriving. Thrivival is where we want to be. It means that thriving is your baseline. It's the minimum you expect from your life.

Your new BMI is about a Better Me Index through Breath, Movement, and Intake. Intake is simply what you eat and what you think.

Before you think this is just another diet or wellness book, I need to introduce you to the concept of the Secret Formula that changes everything. The Secret Formula is about YOU,

Think of each day as a buffet in front of you. Endless food choices, activities, and responses to stimuli are offered throughout your day. How do you know which one works for

YOU, based on your unique base constitution and minor imbalances you might be experiencing?

Imagine knowing exactly what choice to make in each moment. That's your Secret Formula, and we'll get to the details. At the end of the book, you'll find your You Playbook, which will walk you through discovering the elements of your unique body, and how to choose the right B(reath), M(ovement) and I(ntake) for you.

I also made you a more comprehensive You Playbook that you can get separately if you like to have more room to keep notes. Future You will enjoy reading how you got there.

Right now, you're probably tempted to jump to the back of the book and look at the You Playbook section. You can do that, but you'll get a lot more out of it if you wait until you understand the framework better.

If you must jump ahead - it's okay. Just circle back here to know how to use the You Playbook.

Medicine is advancing- we need to participate!

The advances in medicine are extraordinary, and Western medicine is miraculous regarding acute medical problems. Chronic disease, which is endemic in our society, is where we spend most of our healthcare dollars. We spend 4 trillion dollars ANNUALLY in health care in the U.S. That's a lot of money that could be used elsewhere!

Using traditional medicine to drive peak wellness and modern medicine to overcome acute and unavoidable conditions is a winning combo. It's chocolate and peanut butter 10x. It's the best of two extraordinary and efficacious systems.

Imagine how Future You can thrive with access to all the tools you need to stay in peak condition regardless of your age, AND the best that modern medicine offers! As we take control over our wellness and reduce the dollars spent on chronic diseases, we free up resources to work on better treatments for unavoidable health problems.

What would happen to your health and the health of the people you love if an extra trillion dollars or so a year went towards age-reversal medicine and systems to help the entire planet thrive?

How often have you had the chance to participate in an activity that could help save the country you live in trillions of dollars? That's precisely what we can do by reducing chronic diseases! Current You really *is* a superhero!

If we can reduce chronic diseases, we can increase health spans and quality of life and greatly impact our future. Estimates are that we spend 70-80% of our healthcare dollars on chronic diseases. The financial gain to individual budgets and Medicaid/Medicare spending would be impressive if we could reduce chronic disease by even 10%.

Future You really wants more of that money in their pocket. They have plans and goals, and that money will help them reach them. Now is a good time to close your eyes again and connect with Future You. How are you going to spend that money? Travel? Education? Family? Future You wants to know that you'll do everything you can to avoid the following problems:

Chronic diseases, called non-communicable diseases, have risen in the United States over the past century. These diseases include heart disease, cancer, chronic respiratory diseases, diabetes, and other long-term illnesses.

Your doctor can help you manage chronic disease. But doctors aren't in your body. They cannot make the necessary changes to help you reverse and possibly eliminate chronic disease in your body. That is up to you. Understanding the mechanisms behind chronic diseases and helping you avoid them completely will give you power over your vibrant wellness.

Think about it like a car. Have you ever had a noise from your car that was intermittent? I did. It drove me crazy! I took it to the mechanic three times, and three times, the noise did not happen. He finally suggested that we trade cars for a couple of days. It worked! On the second day, he heard the noise, figured it out, and fixed it.

Unfortunately, your doctor can't switch bodies with you. Nobody knows your body like you do. There are simple things you do to your car, like washing it and giving it gas, that are required regularly.

You don't go to your mechanic whenever you need gas or window washing. Learning to do the basics to fuel and protect your body is empowering. But first, you must know what kind of car you're driving.

I had a friend who drove a diesel car in the 90s. Diesel cars weren't common then, and very few people had them. She lent her car to a coworker who had a minor crisis, and I think you can guess what happened next. The coworker, of course, wanted to show her gratitude by filling up the car. She filled it with gas instead of diesel and created a big problem.

So, are you a gas engine or a diesel? High test, regular? With humans, it's a lot more complex. Think of each of us having a specialized blend that makes us run optimally and gives us incredible mileage. Wouldn't finding out what your blend is be a powerful tool? In other words, there is no magic pill you can take, but there is a Secret Formula and finding that changes everything.

The solution is to take what we know to be common sense and use the techniques used for thousands of years to manage wellness successfully. Creating customized health that works for you is easier than ever. You can find your Secret Formula. To paraphrase from a classic TV show (Bionic Man), Future You can be better than you were before- better, stronger, faster.

MAP YOUR FUTURE:

The real you isn't the person struggling through the day or the week, battling fatigue, and living the life that seems pre-scripted. The real you is creative, enthusiastic, and deeply engaged in living a great life.

How do you find the real you? You find the Secret Formula, the special blend that makes you operate at peak efficiency.

Most of us are chronically unhealthy. This robs us of motivation, creativity, and energy. When you uncover the real you through peak wellness, you uncover abilities and motivations you don't know you have. Things you didn't think you were capable of become your baseline. You become as extraordinary as the times we are in.

We are shaping the future of humanity as we maneuver through exponentially world-changing challenges we are facing. We can turn away and pretend it isn't happening, or we can rise to the challenge of these times by becoming the best version of ourselves.

You are far more than you think you are. You are more intelligent, happier, and valuable than you can see now. You aren't living the epic life you came here to live because you haven't been given the tools to be the most potent version of yourself. Future You is astounding, and I can't wait to meet them!

You're about to change all of that. You're about to learn how to create the special Secret Formula that takes you to the best version of yourself.

What is your Secret Formula? It is a personalized plan of different Breathing techniques, Movements, and Intake that work for you—your new BMI. There is a way of understanding who you are at your most elemental level and using that understanding to fill your toolbox with the right tools to hone you to peak health.

We're using methods that come from ancient wisdom and have served to keep humans healthy long before our modern world introduced the variables that led us astray.

You'll use your You Playbook to know which tool to use at which time. You'll understand what works and see results. More importantly, your You Playbook will lead you to find things you enjoy doing. Instead of a journey of deprivation and hardship, you can have a journey full of delicious foods, fun activities, and the conscious creation of your state of being. Sounds good?

Chapter 3

Chapter 3: Our Bright Future!

Real wellness is a vibrancy that we feel. We connect to our bodies and minds, creating a constant feedback loop. We don't need a test to tell us when something is right or wrong. We feel it. Natural wellness has us waking up eager to start our day. We're engaged in the world in positive and productive ways that make us happy and healthy. We've lost touch with this ability, but it awaits us.

I'm not saying there isn't a place for testing and measuring what is happening in our bodies or for conventional medicine. It should be where we go when we know something isn't right and we've done everything we can do with lifestyle choices.

When we marry our commitment to our well-being with the tools available through modern medicine, we create a level of wellness and longevity that changes everything. When you look at the Blue Zones, where people regularly live into their late nineties and even into their hundreds while living full, independent lives, you can see that it is not only possible but probable if you do the things that work for you.

Our overreliance on tests and pills was an easy trap to fall into and completely understandable. When antibiotics, anesthesia, and pain medication emerged, millions of lives were saved, and untold suffering was abated.

We went from a world where limbs were sawed off with nothing but a rag to bite on and people could die from a superficial infection to a world of medical miracles that kept expanding.

At the same time, society and our food supply industrialized, and the beginnings of sedentary lifestyles and repetitive movements emerged. We went from a world where people ate whole foods and lived active lifestyles to a world that has become increasingly toxic and has limited access to the organic, whole foods of 100 years ago.

We call eating right, exercising, and other good habits "lifestyle choices." This isn't accurate. For many of us, it isn't about choice. It's about availability and real knowledge and tools to make it happen.

Am I just my body?

I have a personal dislike for the metric known as BMI—Body Mass Index. My mother struggled with her weight her entire life. She had a goal weight based on BMI, but it was never realistic. Had she understood who she was and her own Secret Formula, her life would have been much different.

The BMI chart tells you whether you're considered "fat." It is what a doctor will use to say to you that you are considered overweight. It's one of the many metrics that take a single measure, usually out of context, and ascribe a more significant value to the metric than what might be true.

This book will turn that one disempowering, discouraging acronym into an empowering, uplifting one. I want you to have a map to experiencing your vibrant wellness based on who you are and what *you need*. Your new BMI-your Better Me Index gives you tools and feedback that work through Breath, Movement, and Intake. They are the toolboxes from which you will pick specific tools that work for your unique body. First, let's talk about how we measure wellness.

Living a great life!

We know what the fundamental metrics of a good life are. Joy, gratitude, strong relationships, and a sense of purpose are all powerful indicators of a good life. Perhaps a great life. Our connection to the natural world also measures how well our life goes.

There are thousands of books on diet, exercise, and wellness. More get published every day. People are seeking a deeper understanding of achieving natural health.

Most people face the challenge that doing the "right" thing isn't as fun as doing the "wrong" thing. Ice cream and French fries are more fun than carrot sticks and celery.

The notion that deprivation is the key to health is wrong. Until we change the frame and find satisfaction in the right choices, we'll continue to get caught in the loop of bad habits, creating bad feelings in our body and mind and using those bad habits to help us feel temporarily better. After we indulge, we generally feel worse and vow to stop doing that. Until the next time...

It's the same with "exercise." For many, that word brings up a sense of obligation and sometimes dread. We force ourselves to do it. What about play? Remember play? Did anyone ever have to force you to play? If we design lives that include activities that create the same effect as "exercise," isn't that a better way to live our lives?

People choose to play over exercise in most cases. That is why pickleball is such a phenomenon. It's about how it is framed and how you choose to experience it.

You're in charge!

The problem with the myriad information on how we should eat, exercise, and live our lives is that it focuses on trying to teach us something that works for some. Nothing works for everyone. You have to know what works for you. You have to be able to mix your Special Formula.

When you pick up a book or listen to a podcast, and people are talking about this "thing" that was so transformational for them and others, and you try it, and it doesn't work, it can be deeply discouraging. The problem isn't the "thing." It's that it wasn't the right thing for you.

You are a complex individual. Unless you are an identical twin, no one is like you. Wouldn't it be great if someone could wave a wand and tell you how to eat, exercise, and sleep to become the peak version of yourself? Not what works for others, but the things that work specifically for you, based on thousands of years of data?

How empowering would it be if you could self-diagnose minor imbalances in yourself and know how to correct those with easy lifestyle tweaks?

This book will guide you to understand what works for you in all aspects of your wellness. Some people thrive as vegans, some as carnivores, and others thrive by diet restrictions. Some people stumble upon what works for them early in life; others struggle their whole lives and never find it.

Finding out what works for you will change everything. The new BMI framework is about Breath, Movement, and Intake – the triangle of wellness that has been successful for as long as humans have been on this planet.

Discovering what works for you within all the myriad variations in that wellness triangle is the key.

Chapter 4

Why BMI?

The old BMII is a bellwether for how we look at many things today.

Instead of a holistic view, we look at parts and pieces and reach conclusions that might be negated if all the data were considered. In seeking metrics we can use in all cases, we've closed our eyes to the more comprehensive view.

Using the BMI acronym to help us understand and practice wellness holistically reminds us that single metrics aren't meant to show us a comprehensive picture. It's good to remember this in all aspects of our lives. For many people, the Body Mass Index was a painful thing.

The Body Mass Index (BMI) is a widely used method for assessing whether an individual has a healthy weight or is overweight. It was developed as a simple statistical tool to measure body fatness and determine potential health risks associated with weight. However, while BMI is a commonly used measurement, it has limitations and can have psychological implications, particularly regarding self-esteem, especially in women.

The concept of BMI originated in the mid-19th century when Adolphe Quetelet, a Belgian mathematician, sought to develop a formula to assess body composition. He proposed using an individual's weight divided by the square of their height, resulting in the calculation known as BMI. Quetelet intended to develop a population-level measure rather than an individual diagnostic tool. Over time, BMI gained popularity as a simple and cost-effective method for assessing weight status. We began using it as a separate metric despite never being intended to be that.

To calculate BMI, an individual's weight in kilograms is divided by the square of their height in meters (BMI = weight/$(\text{height})^2$). The resulting number is then categorized into different ranges to indicate weight status. The World Health Organization (WHO) and many national health agencies typically use the following categories:

Underweight: BMI less than 18.5

Normal weight: BMI between 18.5 and 24.9

Overweight: BMI between 25 and 29.9

Obesity: BMI of 30 or higher, further divided into Class I (30-34.9), Class II (35-39.9), and Class III (40 or higher)

BMI provides a general indication of weight status and potential health risks associated with weight. It is frequently used in epidemiological research and clinical settings to evaluate population health trends and guide interventions. However, it is essential to recognize that BMI does not directly measure body fat percentage, muscle mass, or distribution of fat in the body. As a result, it may not accurately reflect an individual's overall health or risk for certain health conditions.

BMI as a measure of weight status has raised concerns about its potential psychological impact, particularly on self-esteem, body image, and body dissatisfaction, primarily among women. Society's emphasis on thinness as an ideal beauty standard has contributed to the adverse effects of using BMI to evaluate attractiveness and self-worth. The overreliance on BMI as a sole indicator of health can lead to a narrow focus on weight and shape, leading to body dissatisfaction, disordered eating behaviors, and low self-esteem.

Women, in particular, may face societal pressures to conform to unrealistic standards of thinness. BMI in healthcare, media, and personal relationships can reinforce these unrealistic ideals, contributing to negative self-perception and body image issues. The emphasis on BMI and weight can overshadow other important aspects of health, such as mental well-being, physical fitness, and overall quality of life.

It is crucial to recognize that health is multifaceted and cannot be accurately determined by a single measure like BMI. Promoting a holistic approach to health that includes physical activity, nutrition, mental well-being, and body positivity is essential for supporting individuals in developing healthy relationships with their bodies.

In recent years, there has been growing criticism and recognition of the limitations of the Body Mass Index (BMI) as a sole indicator of health and body composition. While it has been historically employed as a screening tool for weight-related health risks, there are several reasons why it is considered somewhat problematic and may not provide a comprehensive understanding of an individual's health.

One of the primary concerns with the BMI is that it needs to differentiate between different body types and compositions. It solely considers height and weight, disregarding muscle mass, bone density, and body fat distribution. As a result, individuals with higher muscle mass, such as athletes or individuals who engage in strength training, may have a higher BMI despite being in good physical condition and having lower body fat. On the other hand, older adults or individuals with certain health conditions may have lower muscle mass and higher body fat, yet their BMI may fall within the healthy range.

Muscle, in particular, is denser than fat, meaning it takes up less space but weighs more. This can lead to misleading BMI calculations, especially for individuals with a higher proportion of muscle mass. Consequently, the BMI may inaccurately categorize these individuals as overweight or obese when their body composition is healthy.

Moreover, the BMI does not account for body fat distribution, an essential factor in assessing health risks. Research has shown that excess fat around the abdomen (visceral fat) is more strongly associated with an increased risk of chronic diseases, such as cardiovascular disease and type 2 diabetes, compared to fat stored in other areas of the body. However, the BMI does not consider this distinction and treats all body fat equally.

Furthermore, the BMI needs to address differences in body shapes and proportions. Individuals with different body types, such as ectomorphs (lean and slender) or endomorphs (higher body fat and wider frame), may have varying health risks and body compositions that the BMI does not accurately reflect.

The funny thing about that is that the ancient wisdom of traditional health frameworks has always understood that different body types have different compositions, which relates to many other propensities that can be explored based on the body frame.

Bye-bye, old BMI. Hello, new BMI!

In my practice as a wellness consultant, I see so many people in their thirties, forties, and fifties that are suffering tremendously. You don't have to be one of those. As you declare your new BMI, learn about Breath, Movement, and Intake (what we eat and think). We'll use each of those letters to lead us to true, vibrant wellness.

Chapter 5

Understanding messages from the body

You should know more about the body, and how distilling body type to one metric missed an opportunity for us all to look at ourselves in the mirror and know a lot about our health and what imbalances we might be experiencing.

Body is what we all have; unless we're feeling sick or having problems with our bodies, we take it for granted. We focus primarily on the externalities. What do I look like? How are other people perceiving me? Do they find me attractive? Do they see me as healthy, or are they judging my body?

In my generation, it was, "Does my butt look too big in these pants?" Now it's "Does my butt look big enough in these pants?" Small butts and big breasts were the body fad of my generation. Now big butts and small breasts are in fashion. Body fads are just that: fads. We're not going to live our lives according to fads any longer.

I watched my mother struggle with diet fads and exercise her whole life, feeling like her body wasn't good enough. As a child watching that, the message was clear. There was only one acceptable body type, and you weren't worthy unless you could achieve that look.

When you explore how traditional medicine in different cultures looked at the body, it was very, very different from how we look at it today. Traditional medicine used the body's appearance to help the practitioner and the patient understand how their body type pointed to other likely predispositions.

Your body's size, shape, and natural movements are all clues to your base constitution. Your base constitution is more than how you look. It is also how you are meant to express yourself physically, emotionally, spiritually, and intellectually.

When we boiled it all down to a single metric of mass, it was like trying to create an orchestra from just one musical instrument. A plethora of information that came with the body type was left unexplored.

The base constitution is your specific, unique blend. Your unique blend will have some tendencies that are good and some that may not be as desirable. Keeping yourself in balance based on your knowledge of your base constitution is how you express the highest form of yourself.

Don't worry if you're getting a bit confused. Your You Playbook will unveil your base constitution and help you understand how to ferret out and correct imbalances. There's a system to figure that out, and it's been used for thousands of years.

Each traditional medicine modality looks at it differently. I want to focus on the many commonalities in all these traditions.

Your body is unique; nothing you can do will alter your base constitution. If you are slender and small-boned, you aren't going to wake up one day and be taller or have bigger bones. If your body type means you have a large frame, you won't wake up one day and fit into petite clothes. Who you are is wonderful; celebrate that!

It is key to understand that your body type, whatever it is, has strengths and weaknesses. Knowing what they are helps you to lean into your propensities in a way that creates positive change.

The most important thing to remember is that peak health can look very different in different bodies. Slim does not always equate to healthy, and a little extra weight does not always equate to unhealthy.

If you look at all the traditional systems of understanding the human body, they all look at the height and weight of a person within a total picture. Traditional medicine uses a person's appearance, including body size and type, to help determine base constitution.

You are many things together in a unique balance

Traditional medicines classify body types based on the elements like fire, air, earth, etc. The most well-known is Ayurvedic medicine. Ayurveda is the traditional medicine practiced in India for over 3000 years.

They define body types by Dosha. Dosha speaks to the kind of body you have and points you toward what your unique formula might be based on the elements. In TCM (Traditional Chinese Medicine), they also use the elements, although there are slight differences in their chosen elements.

The Physiomedicalists also worked with the framework of the elements. This framework lets you understand your base constitution, imbalances, and strengths and weaknesses.

Our framework will use fire, water, earth, air, and ether. Each one of these elements has observable characteristics and feels intuitive in our world.

To give you some idea of how these elements might appear in people. we can look at tendencies and imbalances. Fire people are passionate, Water people tend to be more emotional, Ether people are more logic-based, Air people think a lot, and Earth people are more grounded.

You'll find a detailed analysis of each element, along with signs of excess or deficiencies and ways to correct those, in the back of the book in your You Playbook. For now, I just want you to know about these elements and start thinking of how they appear in how we speak about people's personalities, emotions, and illnesses.

Start paying attention to how the elements appear in the world around you. Do you have a favorite season/temperature? Do you love humidity or hate it?

Look at some of the things we say:

- "She's all fired up!" - Fire -
- "Turn off the waterworks." -Water
- "What an airhead!"- Air
- "They are so grounded." - Earth
- "What they said was cold!" -Ether

Looking at the body from the perspective of the elements gives us a framework to understand some of our imbalances and how to use our understanding of elements to rebalance.

Too much fire can be balanced by adding earth, water, or ether. Earth can ground wind, soak up water, or smother the fire. Can you see the patterns?

Here are the five elements described by Ayurveda:

Akasha (Space or Ether): It is associated with hollow or empty places in the body, such as tubes, channels, and the spaces within cells. Akasha is believed to be the source of all matter and represents the capacity for expansion and spaciousness. It's linked to the sense of hearing and the organ of the ear.

Vayu (Air): This represents all forces and movements. It signifies motion, direction, and force and is associated with the sense of touch and the skin. The body is connected with the respiratory system and breathing process.

Tejas or Agni (Fire): This element is associated with the transformative force. It governs metabolism, digestion, and intelligence. Agni is connected to vision and the eyes. It is responsible for maintaining the body temperature and the digestion and absorption of food.

Jala (Water): Jala represents liquidity, cohesiveness, and the aspect of flow in our bodies. It's associated with the sense of taste and tongue organ. It governs all bodily fluids, like blood, lymph, and other secretions.

Prithvi (Earth): This element signifies solidity, stability, and nourishment. It represents the body's physical structure, bones, muscles, and tissues. It's associated with the sense of smell and nose.

Understanding your body type through the lens of the elements gives you an easy framework to manage your wellness. The Ayurvedic dosha system is an easy way to understand the elements in the body.

Here is an overview of the three doshas:

Vata Dosha: Vata is associated with air and space elements. It governs movement, communication, and creativity. Individuals with a dominant Vata Dosha tend to have a slender frame, light body weight, and restless nature. Vata imbalance can manifest as anxiety, dryness, digestive issues, and difficulty getting or staying asleep.

In balance, the Vata Dosha gives us creative, spiritual, and quick-thinking people.

Pitta Dosha: Pitta is linked to the elements of fire and water. It governs metabolism, digestion, and transformation.

Those with a dominant Pitta dosha usually have a medium build, good muscle tone, and a strong appetite for food and intellectual stimulation. Pitta imbalance may lead to anger, inflammation, and excessive heat in the body.

In balance, the Pitta dosha gives us the "get er done" kind of people. They are effective at leadership and can be great project managers.

Kapha Dosha: Kapha relates to water and earth elements. It governs stability, lubrication, and structure. Individuals with a dominant Kapha dosha often have a solid, sturdy build, well-developed muscles, and a tendency to retain weight. Kapha imbalance can manifest as sluggishness, congestion, and emotional attachment.

In balance, the Kapha dosha gives us calm, stable, and capable people. They are the strongest of the doshas and are great listeners. If you need a warm hug, find a Kapha friend!

In Traditional Chinese Medicine, we see the same pattern of identifying qualities associated with body frame types. It also uses elements, although the elements are slightly different. TCM defines constitutions based on the balance of Yin and Yang energies and the relative strength of specific organ systems within an individual.

One commonly used framework in TCM is the classification of constitutions into the following categories:

Yin Constitution: Individuals with a Yin constitution are believed to have a relatively more robust Yin energy than Yang. They may exhibit characteristics such as a slender build, sensitivity to cold, and calm and introverted nature. Yin constitution is associated with the water and earth elements.

Yang Constitution: Those with a Yang constitution have a relatively more robust Yang energy than Yin. They may have a more muscular physique, intolerance to heat, and a more outgoing and active nature. Yang's constitution is associated with fire and air elements.

Balanced Constitution: A balanced constitution indicates a harmonious equilibrium between Yin and Yang energies. Individuals with this type of constitution typically have good overall health, a stable body weight, and balanced emotional tendencies.

It's important to note that these TCM constitutional classifications are not solely based on physical appearance but also consider various factors, including individual symptoms, personality traits, and overall health patterns. TCM practitioners evaluate these factors through pulse diagnosis, observation, and patient history to determine a person's constitutional type.

TCM constitutional types provide insights into an individual's inherent strengths, weaknesses, and potential imbalances. This information helps guide TCM treatment approaches, including herbal medicine, acupuncture, dietary recommendations, and lifestyle adjustments, to restore balance and promote optimal health for each individual based on their constitutional framework.

Physiomedicalists, also known as Eclectic physicians, were a group of 19th-century American physicians who combined aspects of European medical traditions, including Galenic medicine, herbalism, and indigenous healing practices. They had their perspective on constitutions, which differed from traditional Chinese medicine (TCM) or Ayurveda.

In physiomedicalism, constitutions were viewed as a combination of physical and energetic characteristics influencing an individual's overall health and predisposition to specific diseases. Physiomedicalists believed each person had a unique constitutional makeup that determined their response to various treatments and interventions.

Physiomedicalists also used elements in the body, describing the individual's temperature and moistness.

Physiomedicalists categorized constitutions primarily based on four temperaments: sanguine, choleric, melancholic, and phlegmatic. These temperaments were associated with different physiological and psychological traits:

Sanguine: The sanguine temperament was characterized by warmth, enthusiasm, and a tendency toward a robust and healthy constitution. These individuals were believed to have well-balanced bodily fluids and good circulation.

Choleric: Choleric individuals were described as energetic, ambitious, and prone to being hot-tempered. Physiomedicalists associate the choleric temperament with excess heat and an overactive metabolism.

Melancholic: The melancholic temperament was associated with introversion, sensitivity, and a tendency toward melancholy or depression. Physiomedicalists believed these individuals had a more delicate constitution and were prone to imbalances in their vital fluids.

Phlegmatic: Phlegmatic individuals were described as calm, easygoing, and stable. Physiomedicalists associated this temperament with a cooler and moister constitution.

Physiomedicalists recognized that each person had a unique combination of these temperaments, and an individual's constitutional type influenced their susceptibility to certain diseases, preferred treatment modalities, and even dietary recommendations.

Based on their understanding of constitutions, physiomedicalists aimed to customize treatments and therapies to suit each individual's unique makeup. They utilized a combination of herbal remedies, dietary modifications, hydrotherapy, and other natural interventions to restore balance and promote health in their patients, considering each individual's constitutional characteristics and tendencies.

What works, works!

Medicine throughout the ages and different cultures all accepted that the underlying constitution or elements of the person being treated were a key component of how that person should be treated.

Woven through all the traditions is the understanding that body type points to other tendencies and is a shortcut to understanding what a person might need to create vibrant health. When we lost this framework, we lost a lot.

Today, if you line up 100 people diagnosed with the same illness, conventional medicine would likely treat them all the same. Traditional medicines would not.

When I was in school, we were taught that there were three body types: ectomorph, mesomorph, and endomorph, primarily emphasizing the size of a person's frame. It wasn't presented as a way of understanding how to embrace and manage these qualities.

We lose vital information without understanding how your base constitution influences everything else. Since our base constitution informs us of which foods, activities, thoughts, and breathing patterns are best for us, we are just guessing without this knowledge.

Can we conduct a symphony without any players having access to the music? Can we write a book without knowing words? Can we put together an Ikea piece without seeing the instructions? Well, maybe you can do the last one. I can't put them together even with instructions!!

We are viewed as having parts that can be replaced. When something goes wrong in part of our body, it is treated primarily based on that specific symptom, with lesser regard for the total body.

Most interventions are drug-based, and lifestyle changes are usually relegated to sending people home with a paper sheet telling them what they should and shouldn't eat.

I want to applaud conventional medicine for the many ways it recognizes alternative medicine's value. Conventional and "alternative" medicine have been dating for a long time. It's time for them to make a commitment. They each bring something really valuable to the partnership.

Traditional or alternative medicine (I find these terms almost interchangeable) has been flirting with conventional for a long time. They batted eyelashes and whispered "You complete me" to each other for a long time. The truth is, they do each complete the other.

Think of it from a financial standpoint. You have to have your budget for the day-to-day life. That's your daily wellness stuff. You also need to have plans for emergencies. That's your conventional medicine.

If you take care of the budget, then the long-term stuff is easier. If you don't care for the budget, you deplete your emergency fund before it starts. That puts you perpetually behind. The same thing happens with your wellness. Take care of the day-to-day stuff, and you may never need to rely on conventional medicine for emergency care.

By embracing a holistic perspective, we can acknowledge the many qualities that contribute to our individuality, such as our energy levels, metabolism, resilience, personalities, and emotional tendencies. We can finally get real health care.

Imagine how differently we can experience life if we see ourselves and others through the lens of holism. We can all be active participants in creating our joyful lives when we understand how to manage our health and emotional states based on our unique properties.

If we expand our understanding of our body and how it connects to our greater life experience, we have control over our lives. By understanding the elements, strengths, and weaknesses of our particular body type, we can manage our wellness in a way impossible without this knowledge.

How do you apply this knowledge to your life? The way to start is to understand what body type you are. In your You Playbook, we have a questionnaire to help you find your base element(s) and potential imbalances. All five elements are in our makeup, but one or two will be primary.

Reading through the whole book before you go to the You Playbook part will be most helpful, but you can skip to the back if you really need to know. ◈

Understanding what elements you are working with gives you the information to know what tools you can have in your toolbox and how to use them. One of the quickest and easiest tools is the one we'll talk about next. It's free; you can do it anywhere, and it works!

Chapter 6

The B for the new BMI stands for Breath

One of the first tools for managing the body is the breath. We've all probably heard things like "take a deep breath and count to ten" or "calm down and just breathe," but do we understand the power of the breath?

Our body understands and intuitively breathes differently in different situations to help alter the way our body responds to different situations. We pant, sigh, hold our breath, or take a deep breath in response to stimuli.

We can use the breath consciously to alter how our body responds to stimuli, create energy and remove blockages, calm and sedate our nervous system, and so much more. We're going to explore that deeply.

Breath is free and a tool that anyone can learn to use. It gives you immediate access to a method of changing your state. It can be used to slow or speed up your heart rate. Simple breathing techniques can calm the mind, energize the body, and more.

These tools have been underestimated. Conscious breathing is practiced during specific times like a yoga class or a meditation, but how often are we using our breath to help us sleep, manage anxiety, or balance our minds? Implementing this tool also trains the body to make permanent changes in responding to stimuli.

Take a deep breath!

Breathwork is a powerful practice that can profoundly impact the human body and mind. Through various breathing techniques, individuals can alter their state of being and experience a wide range of benefits.

As you understand your elements, you'll understand how different breathing techniques work to strengthen, balance, or decrease how the elements show up in your physicality.

For each of us, there will be times when these breathing techniques can be useful. You can read through them here, and I've made YouTube videos of each one so you can practice. You can find them here: https://bit.ly/Flurban. You won't know until you get into your You Playbook which breath is most beneficial for you now, but practicing each one will familiarize you with this part of your toolbox.

Let's explore the effects of different breathing techniques, including breath of fire, alternate nostril breathing, and other methods commonly used to induce specific states.

Breathing is an essential life function, providing oxygen to our cells and removing waste products like carbon dioxide. However, breathwork goes beyond the basic mechanics of respiration. It involves conscious manipulation of breath patterns to influence physical, mental, and emotional states. By deliberately changing how we breathe, we can access a variety of physiological responses that can positively impact our well-being.

One popular technique is the breath of fire. It is an energizing and invigorating practice involving rapid, rhythmic nose breathing. This technique increases oxygenation, stimulates the sympathetic nervous system, and generates heat.

Breath of fire can enhance alertness, improve mental clarity, and boost overall vitality. It is often used in yoga and meditation to awaken dormant energy, increase focus, and promote a sense of inner strength.

I think we all know what element is at play with breath of fire. When might it be helpful? If you're feeling cold or damp (ether/water). Low energy can be seen as a lack of fire, and breath of fire energizes.

It's not just for having babies!

Imagine practicing breath of fire before your morning coffee or maybe in place of it. It's powerful to energize your body naturally while simultaneously creating deep wellness.

Another technique, alternate nostril breathing, is a balancing and calming practice. It involves alternating the breath between the left and right nostrils by using the fingers to close one nostril at a time gently.

This technique harmonizes the left and right hemispheres of the brain, promoting a sense of equilibrium and mental clarity. Alternate nostril breathing reduces stress, anxiety, and insomnia while enhancing concentration and overall emotional well-being.

The left nostril is associated with the yin aspects. Yin aspects are cooling, relaxing, and cultivating patience. Breathing exclusively through the left nostril can help with anxiety. This technique can help ground excess air and cool too much fire.

Unlike medication, breathing techniques train the body to default to the desired state when the breathing is conscious. Much like Pavlov's dogs, we can train our nervous system to respond to our breathing patterns so quickly that even the first breath changes our state.

The right nostril is associated with yang aspects. Yang's aspects are heating, energizing, and cultivating a desire for action. This can be helpful when we are stuck or a little depressed, or even just to warm up the body. It cultivates fire and can help dissipate excess water.

A great way to start breathing practices is to notice which nostril dominates your breathing at any time. Also, be aware of where the breath is going. Is it deep, slow, and steady? Are you breathing quickly and shallowly? Even simple awareness can change your state.

You can create new, healthier patterns if you become aware of your breathing patterns and how they relate to your emotional and physical state. You're going to breathe every minute for the rest of your life. A little awareness can go a long way toward making those breaths optimum for who you are.

If you are new to breathwork, I encourage you to breathe with some videos to hone your technique. Having someone talking and cueing you when to inhale or exhale is helpful. It enables you to leave everything behind and breathe. This is a powerful way to reset your body, mind, and breath.

Numerous other breathing techniques can induce specific states of being. One such example is the 4-7-8 breathing method, which involves inhaling for a count of four, holding the breath for a count of seven, and exhaling for a count of eight.

This technique, popularized by Dr. Andrew Weil, activates the body's relaxation response, slowing the heart rate and calming the mind. It is often a natural remedy for stress, anxiety, and insomnia.

Wim Hof breathing, named after the Dutch extreme athlete Wim Hof, is another notable technique. It involves a series of deep inhalations and forceful exhalations, followed by a period of breath retention. This technique aims to increase oxygen intake, alkalize the body, and elevate energy levels. Wim Hof's breathing is often combined with cold exposure and has been associated with improved immune function, increased tolerance to stress, and enhanced mental resilience.

Breathwork also encompasses practices such as box, belly, and coherent breathing, each with unique effects on the body and mind. Box breathing, also known as square breathing, involves inhaling, holding, exhaling, and holding the breath for equal counts. This technique promotes relaxation, reduces anxiety, and improves focus.

Belly breathing, or diaphragmatic breathing, focuses on deep inhalations that expand the belly, helping to activate the body's natural relaxation response and alleviate tension. Coherent breathing, conversely, involves maintaining a regular inhaled and exhaled rhythm for a specific count, promoting a balanced and cohesive state of being.

Beyond their immediate effects, these breathing techniques can profoundly impact our well-being. Regular breathwork practice has been shown to improve respiratory function, increase lung capacity, and enhance cardiovascular health.

It can also reduce blood pressure, alleviate chronic pain, and boost the immune system. Moreover, breathwork has been recognized for reducing symptoms of anxiety, depression, and post-traumatic stress disorder (PTSD). By regulating our breath, we can tap into the autonomic nervous system and influence our body's physiological responses, leading to improved mental states. Learning to use the simple tools of breathing can change your life!

The practice of breathwork has a rich history spanning various cultures and traditions. Although the specific techniques and purposes may vary, the underlying principle of harnessing the power of breath to enhance well-being remains constant.

How long have we been breathing?

Let's explore the historical roots of breathwork and some examples of its incorporation into daily lives and routines.

Breathwork has been practiced for thousands of years, with roots in ancient civilizations such as India, China, and Egypt. In ancient Indian traditions, breath control, or pranayama, was vital to yoga and meditation.

The Indian sage Patanjali, in his Yoga Sutras, outlined specific techniques for breath control to calm the mind and achieve higher states of consciousness. The concept of prana, or life force energy, is central to these practices, with breath being the primary vehicle for cultivating and directing prana.

In traditional Chinese medicine, breathwork is integral to qigong and tai chi practices. These ancient arts emphasize the cultivation and balance of qi, the vital energy that flows through the body. Qigong exercises incorporate specific breathing techniques to facilitate the smooth flow of qi, improve overall health, and promote mental clarity and emotional well-being.

The incorporation of breathwork can also be seen in various spiritual and religious traditions. For example, in Buddhism, mindfulness of breath is a fundamental practice. Practitioners cultivate present-moment awareness and develop concentration by observing and anchoring attention to the breath. Similarly, in Sufism, a mystical branch of Islam, specific breathing techniques facilitate spiritual awakening and deepen the connection with the divine.

In more recent history, breathwork gained prominence in the West through the work of pioneers such as Wilhelm Reich, Stanislav Grof, and Leonard Orr.

Reich, an Austrian psychoanalyst, explored the connection between breath and emotional well-being, developing a technique known as "vegetotherapy" that involved deep breathing to release emotional blockages.

Grof, a Czech psychiatrist, developed Holotropic Breath-work, which utilizes accelerated and deep breathing to access non-ordinary states of consciousness and facilitate personal transformation.

An American therapist, Orr, introduced Rebirthing Breath-work, which focuses on conscious connected breathing to release suppressed emotions and trauma.

Using what works!

Today, individuals can incorporate breathwork into their daily lives and routines in various ways. Here are some practical examples:

Morning Ritual: Start the day with a few minutes of conscious breathing. Take slow, deep breaths, focusing on expanding the belly and fully exhaling. This practice can promote relaxation and mental clarity and set a positive tone for the day.

Mindful Breaks: Incorporate brief breathwork sessions throughout the day as mini-reset moments. Set a timer for a few minutes, close your eyes, and engage in slow, intentional breathing to reduce stress, increase focus, and recharge.

Exercise and Movement: During physical activities such as yoga, running, or weightlifting, pay attention to your breath. Practice rhythmic breathing, synchronizing your inhales and exhales with specific movements. This can enhance performance, improve coordination, and deepen the mind-body connection.

Before Sleep: Wind down before bed with a calming breathwork practice. Try alternate nostril breathing or the 4-7-8 technique mentioned earlier to induce relaxation, release tension, and promote a restful night's sleep.

Dedicated Breathwork Sessions: Set aside specific times for more extended breathwork sessions, where you can explore different techniques such as breath of fire, Wim Hof breathing, or guided breathwork meditations. These sessions allow a deeper dive into self-exploration, stress reduction, and personal growth.

What's in it for me?

Using breathwork can have a transformative impact on a person's life and health. Here are some examples of how breathwork can bring about positive changes:

Stress Reduction: Breathwork techniques activate the parasympathetic nervous system, promoting relaxation and reducing the effects of stress. By incorporating breathwork into daily life, individuals can experience lower levels of stress, improved emotional well-being, and enhanced resilience in the face of challenges.

Improved Mental Clarity: Certain breathwork practices, such as alternate nostril breathing or coherent breathing, help balance brain hemispheres and increase oxygenation to the brain. This can improve mental focus, clarity, and enhanced cognitive function.

Emotional Regulation: Breathwork provides a powerful tool for emotional regulation and self-awareness. By consciously regulating their breath, individuals can access and release suppressed emotions, reduce anxiety, and cultivate a greater sense of emotional balance and well-being.

Enhanced Energy and Vitality: Breathwork techniques like breath of fire or Wim Hof breathing stimulate energy systems, increase oxygen intake, and alkalize the body. This can result in heightened energy levels, increased vitality, and improved physical performance.

Boosted Immune Function: Deep, diaphragmatic breathing and certain breathwork practices have positively influenced immune function. By increasing oxygenation and facilitating better circulation, breathwork can support the immune system, improving health and resilience.

Improved Respiratory Function: Regular breathwork strengthens respiratory muscles, increases lung capacity, and enhances overall respiratory function. This can benefit individuals with respiratory conditions such as asthma or chronic obstructive pulmonary disease (COPD).

Enhanced Emotional Well-being: Breathwork can profoundly impact mental and emotional well-being. By consciously manipulating the breath, individuals can release emotional blockages, reduce symptoms of anxiety and depression, improve self-awareness, and cultivate a greater sense of inner peace and happiness.

Better Sleep: Incorporating breathwork techniques before bedtime can help promote relaxation and improve sleep quality. By engaging in calming breathing practices, individuals can quiet the mind, release tension, and establish a more peaceful state conducive to a restful night's sleep.

Increased Mind-Body Connection: Breathwork practices deepen the connection between the mind and body, facilitating greater self-awareness and embodiment. This heightened mind-body connection can improve physical coordination, greater intuitive insight, and a deeper understanding of one's needs and well-being.

Transformation and Personal Growth: Breathwork can be a powerful personal transformation and self-discovery tool. By accessing altered states of consciousness through specific breathwork techniques, individuals may gain profound insights, release trauma, and experience profound shifts in their perspectives and beliefs, leading to personal growth and self-empowerment.

Fun fact: If you're trying to achieve orgasm and just can't seem to get there, it might be that your body needs a little more oxygen. Breath of fire can help get oxygen where it's needed. If it's because you're too much in your head, the act of conscious breathing takes you out of your head. You're welcome. Wink.

Finding your best breath

Breathwork is a tool you can use anytime, anywhere. As you give yourself the gift of learning and using this powerful tool, you also provide yourself with control over your present and future wellness. Using breath to manage the body empowers you to be the master of your state and your fate.

Now that you have all these tools, which is for you? All these breathing methods will likely be helpful at different times. To find the breathing techniques that work for you, let's explore you.

Do you wake up full of energy and ready to start your day? Or do you wake up foggy and have trouble getting moving? The Breath of Fire technique will help. Two to three minutes of Breath of Fire will increase your energy levels and help oxygen get deep into your tissues. It will also help wake your digestive system and give your internal organs a little morning massage. You'll see some great benefits from this simple practice.

Are you an anxious person? Do you tend to get stressed easily? Alternate nostril breathing or belly breathing techniques will help calm your nervous system. Not only will it help at the moment, but it also will build resilience in your nervous system.

Is focus something that you struggle with? Box breathing, or any other technique that requires counting the length of the breath, will help to calm and focus a scattered or busy brain.

Take some time to try the different techniques. Observe how they affect you physically, emotionally, and mentally. You'll have valuable tools that are free and available anywhere, anytime.

Deep breathing, for me, has been an enormous boon. I use it before public speaking, while waiting for a plane to take off, or to remind myself that my calmness can help someone else stay calm during a conflict or emergency.

The You Playbook will lead you to the breathing techniques for you.

Chapter 7

You got to move it, move it

Humans evolved as creatures on the go. In the earlier parts of our existence, life naturally contained what we now refer to as cardio, weight training, and stretching. Life wasn't a series of repetitive movements. It was active and intense. Our days consisted of walking, running, bending, climbing, pulling, etc.

Agriculture changed everything. Our wildly diverse diets became more homogenous. Our movements changed, too. Repetition of movement became more common. We were no longer climbing and reaching to harvest fruit or bending, tugging, and digging to get roots from the ground daily. We were doing things like plowing, weeding, and harvesting. It was still a very movement-oriented lifestyle but with less variety of movement.

Exercise has become a negative word for many people. It evokes the idea of mind-numbing, uncomfortable activities. It doesn't have to be that way! I've found substituting the word fun for the word exercise helpful. Try it!

Turn to the person beside you and say, "Hey, let's get some fun today." It isn't grammatically correct, but doesn't it sound fun? If you substitute the word fun for every time you think or say exercise, you'll change how you view it:

"I have to get some fun today."

"I need to incorporate some fun into my routine."

"I'm getting up early tomorrow to go fun."

It won't change your resistance overnight, but it will help. Unless the word exercise invokes nothing but positive imagery, insert the word "fun" instead of the word exercise.

It might inspire you to new activities when you start thinking of movement as fun, not exercise. For example, I've always wanted to join a freeze tag league. I loved freeze tag as a child. Why shouldn't I still play?

We will explore how to make moving our body fun, but first, let's understand the overwhelming body of evidence on how much better life is when you have regular movement in your schedule.

Movement and exercise play a crucial role in human health and well-being. The importance of physical activity is supported by extensive research, and the most recent recommendations emphasize its numerous benefits across different aspects of health.

Even if you know all the benefits of active fun, it's good to review. If you want to look, feel, and age better, exercise ticks all those boxes and more.

Moving towards more joy, more love, more LIFE!

Regular movement and exercise positively impact cardiovascular health, mental well-being, weight management, musculoskeletal strength, and longevity.

Cardiovascular Health: Physical activity has a profound impact on cardiovascular health. Regular exercise helps improve heart function, reduces the risk of heart disease, lowers blood pressure, and improves cholesterol profiles. It enhances the efficiency of the cardiovascular system, leading to better oxygen and nutrient delivery to the body's tissues.

Mental Well-being: Exercise is closely linked to mental health and emotional well-being. It has been shown to reduce symptoms of depression, anxiety, and stress. Regular physical activity promotes the release of endorphins, known as "feel-good" hormones, which can improve mood and alleviate symptoms of mental health disorders. Additionally, exercise can enhance cognitive function, memory, and overall brain health.

Weight Management: Engaging in regular physical activity is essential for weight management. Exercise helps burn calories, increase metabolism, and build lean muscle mass. Combining regular physical activity with a balanced diet can support healthy weight loss, weight maintenance, and the prevention of weight-related conditions such as obesity and type 2 diabetes.

Musculoskeletal Health: Movement and exercise are critical for maintaining strong bones, muscles, and joints. Weight-bearing exercises, resistance training, and activities that promote flexibility and balance help build and preserve bone density, improve muscle strength, and support joint health. Regular exercise can also reduce the risk of age-related conditions like osteoporosis and sarcopenia.

Longevity and Disease Prevention: Research consistently demonstrates that regular physical activity is associated with increased longevity and a reduced risk of chronic diseases. Engaging in moderate-intensity exercise for at least 150 minutes per week or vigorous-intensity exercise for 75 minutes per week, along with muscle-strengthening activities, is recommended by various health organizations. This activity level has been linked to a lower risk of cardiovascular disease, certain cancers, stroke, and type 2 diabetes.

Recent recommendations from organizations like the World Health Organization (WHO) and the American Heart Association (AHA) emphasize the importance of a balanced exercise regimen that combines aerobic activity, strength training, and flexibility exercises. These recommendations also highlight the significance of reducing sedentary behavior and promoting regular daily movement.

Newer research points to the importance of exercise in making the body more sensitive to insulin, helping to manage blood sugar, and reducing damaging insulin spikes.

<u>There are two other points that I'd like to make about movement:</u>

People who move regularly also move more youthfully.

You know the difference. Some people move like they are 40 when they are 80, and others move like they are 80 when they are 40. We're going to be the former. It's not just about how we appear to others. Being able to move easily and freely feels so much better.

People who move regularly have better sex.

Circulation is an important part of a good sex life. I think we all know what good blood flow, or lack of blood flow, can do for our sex organs. Regular movement practices mean better circulation and, therefore, equals better sex. Also, glowing good health makes you more attractive at any age.

What moves you?

The most important key in your movement journey is understanding what form the movement should take to be most beneficial to you. It is also about finding the activity that you love to do. Something that you love to do isn't exercise-it's fun. Don't we want more fun in our lives?

When you're talking about movement, there are aspects that I find interesting. There is the activity you love to do, and there is the activity with the most positive impact on the totality of your being. They are usually two different things, and knowing and including both in your routines is life-changing.

First, the activity that you love to do. We've all met people who can't sit still and others who seem glued to the couch. If you take someone who typically has a slower pace of life and put them into a slow-paced stretching class, they might enjoy it, but is it the best thing for them? Or is it just reinforcing their already slow pace?

I love playing soccer because it's fast-paced, and I'm not thinking about what my body is doing. I'm just having fun, and it's great for the cardio aspect of my movement needs. Is it the best thing for me? Not necessarily. It feeds my already high drive and cultivates aspects of my being that are already strong.

Because it is easy and natural for me to want to engage in more intense activities, soccer can fire me up a little too much. Notice that I said fire me up. The fire element is naturally strong in me. Activities that fire me up can translate into being more aggressive, reactive, and impulsive.

The activity that I've had to cultivate a love for is yoga. It wasn't initially as attractive to me as soccer, but I credit my yoga practice to my being able to still play soccer at 63. It gave me the weight training and stretching I needed but wasn't attracted to in their conventional forms. Yoga offered the challenge that my fierier nature required, but it balanced that fire rather than feeding it.

For many people, the challenge is about getting off the couch. In that case, the first step is to find a fun activity. Doing what is fun for you and getting you to where you can get 150 minutes of movement a week is an important step. These people need to be fired up, so a team sport gets them engaged, and the desire to be a team player helps to motivate them to get up and show up.

Another important thing about your movement journey is to seek as much variety as possible. Many of us have fallen into the trap of routine. We have leg days, cardio days, abs days, etc. We repeat our routine week after week, never exploring the parts of us that may not be getting the attention that we need. This can lead to imbalanced bodies that are overly developed in some areas and underdeveloped in others. Having strong muscles is essential. Having strong AND flexible bodies is how you live a vibrantly healthy life.

Your element test in the workbook will also give ideas on what kind of movement is best for your particular body type or current imbalances. Once you know the kind of physical activity best for you, you can incorporate those while finding other activities you love. Balance is the key.

Another reason that I used the BMI acronym in this work is because it can help us remember what we need to, B- Body, Breath, Balance, Better, M- Movement, Meditation. Mindfulness, Me I- Intake, Intuition, Inspiration, Inner. I hope that you'll create your own interpretation of BMI. Is it Build More Inspiration? Be Mindfully Intuitive? Best Me Index? You decide. It's yours. You own it!

You can buy all the equipment and memberships in the world, but you'll eventually stop if it doesn't engage you. If getting yourself to exercise is a mental wall you must climb every day, sooner or later, you'll avoid that wall.

If exercise is something you turn to manage stress or body wellness naturally, then there isn't a wall to climb. Instead, it becomes a refuge. When it is a fun activity that you look forward to, you don't have to fight yourself to do it.

Making sure I get Moved. Tools for Success

It's counterintuitive to say that the exercise you least like to do is probably the one you need to do the most, especially after all that talk about making it fun. But the key is getting your "want to" routine fired up. Then you tie in the "good for me" in some way. You can use habit stacking to link one activity to the other.

Habit stacking is simply attaching an activity you would like to become a habit to a habit you already have. One activity cues your brain to do the next, making it more accessible. This method, which was created by BJ Fogg as part of his Tiny Habits program,2 and can be used to design an obvious cue for nearly any habit.

I used habit stacking to get yoga into my morning routine by doing it right after walking the dogs. No matter what, I have to walk the dogs daily, so it's a good trigger for me. I walk into the room where I do my yoga every morning. Some days, I'm only in there for 10 minutes, and all I do is lay on the mat.

Most days, I spend 20-30 minutes doing whatever my body feels like doing. The point is to show up. The more you show up consistently, the easier it becomes. Good habits can be just as hard to break as bad ones.

Move me some more! Setting goals and reaching them.

Some key strategies will help you become more successful in transitioning to good habits. One crucial part of goal setting is that you must set the goals. Your goals can't come from someone else or your "should" drawer.

We all have a "should" drawer. I should do this; I shouldn't do that. This is where we put other people's expectations of who we are and how we show up. Throw out everything in your should drawer. Then, sit in your favorite place, go into your heart, and ask yourself what you want for yourself. Set goals around those things.

I love to hike. I've only spent a few nights on the Appalachian Trail but I want to spend much more. To do that, I have to maintain a level of fitness. This is a primary motivation for me.

Watching the children whom I love grow up and being able to run around with them as they grow is another primary motivation. I use my primary motivations to drive the setting of my goals.

Take a moment here and have a chat with Future You. What motivates you now, and what does the Future You want? What will you do in two, five, and ten years, and what movements will you want to do?

While it is never too late to start a movement practice, today is always the best day. Talk to Future You. What will they be looking for from their body? Do they want to coach sports for children or grandchildren? Walk the El Camino? Travel and explore new places?

I will give you an affirmation that will make any changes much easier if you start by repeating it over and over to yourself. Make it the last thing you hear at night and the first thing you think in the morning. "In every moment, I am designing my future and building an amazing future for myself and my loved ones.."

When it's late at night, and you've just eaten some junk food, it is not the best time to set goals for the next day. Chances are, you'll be a little unrealistic. I've gone to bed many nights after convincing myself I'd be up at dawn and do a great workout. It didn't happen. It's easy to imagine that you'll be a peak athlete when you're sitting on the couch. It just isn't realistic.

Setting goals is while you are getting ready to do the activity. You put on your yoga/workout clothes first. You show up and set your goals when it is time to begin achieving them. When you're ready to take that first step, you decide about the journey. It makes it real and helps you set more realistic goals.

The only goal that is good to set while you're on the couch the night before is the goal of just showing up.

Keep me Moving-temptation bundling!

Another good thing to do is to feed your inherent reward system through temptation bundling. This involves tying something you really enjoy to something that you don't enjoy so much. I have a lot of repetitive tasks in my life. Saving my favorite podcasts or shows for the times when I have repetitive tasks makes me look forward to doing the chore.

Sometimes, I save my repetitive chores for when I have company. A friend stops by for a cup of tea or a chat, and I'll put the beans I need to shell on the table or the bananas that need to be peeled to go in the freezer. Sometimes, when my repetitive chores have piled up after a few harvests, it inspires me to invite over a good friend. You can use that same method to increase your movement.

If a friend stops by, it's a great chance to let them inspire you or you inspire them. Let them know that you really feel like going for a bike ride, or a skate, or a jog, or a walk in the park. Turn your social activities active, and you might find more movement bodies and more socializing than you thought!

Remember this: Every time two or more people come together, compromises are made. You'll be more active if you hang out with active people. If you hang out with couch potatoes, you're more likely to be a couch potato.

Temptation bundling is a great way to inspire movement. Love loud music? Use it as a trigger to inspire you to move. Have friends you love to hang out with? Make it a movement.

Scheduling your Me Time is also a great way to inspire routine. I give myself an hour, sometime between 12-2, to read, nap, whatever I want. I follow that with a short swim, bike ride, or something. Just a quick activity, twenty to thirty minutes, to get me back to a place of doing. This gives me a fresh start to the second half of my day.

If you go to a physical location for work, how can you make that part of your day more nourishing for your body? For example, I am writing this at a walking desk. I walk for a couple of hours a day and break it up by sitting for periods. If you work at a desk, how can you incorporate movement?

It can be as simple as taking a couple of laps around the office/building you're in every hour or so. Setting an alarm for this is helpful. Take the stairs. Stand up and stretch. Swing your arms. Talk to your employer about bringing in a yoga class before or after work or for lunch.

Knowing that the activity you don't initially love makes it possible for you to do the other activity that you DO love can be the initial motivation to make it part of the routine. If it's part of the routine, you'll begin to see its impact on your life. It didn't take long to see that Yoga created space for many other good things in my life. It has been crucially beneficial in my aging well journey also.

People who know me are sometimes surprised by my love for VR workouts. I'm a tree-hugging-nature-loving-low waste-grow your food-take care of the planet kind of crunchy person. You wouldn't meet me and think, "I bet this person loves technology." It's more likely that people would view me as a Luddite.

I love VR workouts for the same reason I love soccer. They are fun, fast, and available anytime. These workouts are GREAT for couch people. All you need is the motivation to put on the headset; before you know it, you're having fun. It doesn't feel like exercise. I'm a BIG fan. I like the Supernatural app.

Dance is also a great way to find your movement bliss. It also has an easy on switch, like the VR. Fire up the music that you love, and just move.

As the Queen song says- Don't stop me now!

You already know that movement is essential. If you still can't inspire yourself to move after you've read this book and done the work in the workbook, that signifies a deeper resistance that we can explore.

Did you have a bad experience at some point? Maybe you missed the shot, and the class laughed? Or you were the slowest, and nobody picked you? It's time to put that in the past. You can find a therapist to get you over that. Cognitive Behavior Therapy, Hypnosis, and Rescripting are all ways to move forward.

Another reason a person can have trouble motivating for movement is poor nutrition. You know what you've been eating and not eating, so you'll know the answer to this. It's okay, you don't have to tell us.

We've all had our times when junk food was our best friend. But those days are over. So, if you are struggling with motivation because you just don't feel well, focus first on intake. As you get your intake gets better, you'll begin to have more energy.

If poor nutrition is stealing your energy, then while you are rectifying that, start with just a little more movement than you currently get. Every step is a step forward.

Very few of us are natural athletes. We aren't all great dancers or naturally coordinated. That is not what movement is about. Movement is about creating and maintaining the best vehicle to carry around the amazing human that you are.

Movement is for honing the container that carries all the love, knowledge, talent, and uniqueness you are and giving it the best tools to allow you to be the best version of yourself you have ever been.

In the You Playbook, you'll learn which activities can best serve you based on your base constitution. In the section below, we explore some of those modalities. If you'd like, you can wait and read the section(s) that apply to you.

I recommend reading through it all because knowing which movement practices resonate with you is good. Take note of which are appealing and which are not. Write that down, and write down why or why not. That's good info as you explore your motivations.

There's something for everyone!

Many ancient forms of exercise have been practiced for centuries and continue to be influential today. There is great wisdom in these ancient practices, and if you've never practiced some of them, why not take a class or watch a video and see how they make you feel?

Yoga: Originating in ancient India, yoga is a holistic practice that combines physical postures (asanas), breath control (pranayama), and meditation. It promotes physical strength, flexibility, balance, and mental well-being.

Qigong: Developed in ancient China, Qigong is a system of exercises that combines movement, breath control, and meditation to cultivate and balance the body's vital energy (Qi). It is practiced to enhance overall health, promote relaxation, and support the body's energy flow.

Tai Chi originated in ancient China as a martial art and self-defense system. It has evolved into a gentle exercise emphasizing slow, flowing movements, balance, and internal energy cultivation. Tai Chi is known for its numerous health benefits and is often practiced for physical and mental well-being.

Greek Gymnastics: Ancient Greeks emphasized physical fitness and incorporated exercises and athletic activities into their daily lives. Gymnastics played a vital role in Greek education, including running, jumping, wrestling, and discus throwing.

Chinese Martial Arts (Kung Fu): Various forms of Chinese martial arts, collectively known as Kung Fu, have been practiced for thousands of years. These martial arts systems combine physical movements, self-defense techniques, and mental discipline, promoting physical fitness, self-defense skills, and personal growth.

Indigenous Tribal Rituals and Dances: Many indigenous cultures incorporate ancient forms of exercise into their rituals, dances, and daily practices. These activities often involve rhythmic movements, endurance, and strength-building exercises for physical and spiritual purposes.

These ancient forms of exercise highlight the enduring significance of movement and physical activity for overall health and well-being. They have stood the test of time and continue to be practiced and appreciated for their physical, mental, and spiritual benefits.

Chapter 8

Deeper into movements

Yoga:

Now, we'll go a little deeper into each of these practices. First, yoga. In its many forms, yoga is a beautiful way to manage body wellness holistically. It contains all the elements of our earlier lifestyle: cardio, weight training, and stretching.

Yoga has gained popularity worldwide due to its numerous benefits for the mind, body, and spirit. Incorporating physical postures (asanas), breath control (pranayama), meditation, and ethical principles, yoga offers a range of positive effects on the human body. Some key benefits of practicing yoga are:

Improved Flexibility and Strength: Yoga poses focus on stretching and lengthening the muscles, promoting flexibility, and improving the range of motion. Regular practice can enhance muscle strength, particularly in the core, arms, legs, and back, contributing to better posture and overall physical stability.

Increased Balance and Coordination: Many yoga postures require balance and coordination, which can improve proprioception (awareness of body position) and enhance stability.

Standing poses, balances, and inversions help strengthen the muscles responsible for balance and cultivate a sense of body awareness.

Stress Reduction and Relaxation: Yoga incorporates breathing techniques, meditation, and mindfulness practices, which help activate the body's relaxation response, reducing stress and anxiety. These practices can promote a sense of calmness, improve sleep quality, and enhance overall mental well-being.

Improved Cardiovascular Health: Certain forms of yoga, such as Vinyasa or Power Yoga, involve more vigorous movements and can provide cardiovascular benefits similar to aerobic exercise. Regular yoga practice can improve heart health, lower blood pressure, and reduce the risk of cardiovascular diseases.

Enhanced Respiratory Function: Yoga strongly emphasizes breath control and mindful breathing techniques. Practices like deep diaphragmatic breathing, alternate nostril breathing, and breath awareness can enhance lung capacity, improve respiratory efficiency, and promote overall respiratory health.

Better Body Awareness and Mind-Body Connection: Yoga encourages individuals to cultivate a deeper connection between their body, mind, and breath. Through conscious movement and focused attention, practitioners develop greater body awareness and learn to listen to the body's signals, promoting self-care and overall well-being.

Increased Energy and Vitality: Regular yoga can boost energy levels and improve overall vitality. Combining physical movement, breathwork, and mindfulness helps release tension, invigorate the body, and enhance overall energy flow.

Reduced Chronic Pain: Studies have shown that yoga can benefit individuals with chronic pain conditions such as back pain, arthritis, fibromyalgia, and migraines. Gentle stretching, strengthening exercises, and relaxation techniques in yoga can alleviate pain, improve mobility, and enhance quality of life.

Improved Posture and Spinal Health: Yoga postures focus on spinal alignment and strengthening the supporting muscles, which can help improve posture and reduce the risk of back and neck pain. Regular practice can also promote spinal flexibility and prevent degenerative spinal conditions.

Enhanced Mindfulness and Emotional Well-being: Yoga promotes mindfulness, self-reflection, and emotional balance. It can help individuals develop greater self-awareness, cultivate positive emotions, and manage stress and negative thought patterns more effectively.

It is important to note that yoga is a versatile practice with various styles and intensities. Individuals should choose a style and level of practice that suits their needs and physical abilities. It is advisable to learn yoga under the guidance of a qualified instructor to ensure proper alignment, technique, and safety.

In summary, the practice of yoga offers a multitude of benefits for the human body. From physical strength and flexibility to stress reduction, improved cardiovascular health, and enhanced mindfulness, yoga provides a holistic approach to well-being, promoting harmony between the mind, body, and spirit.

Qigong

Qigong, pronounced "chee-gong," is an ancient Chinese practice that integrates movement, breath control, and meditation to cultivate and balance the body's vital energy, known as Qi (or Chi). It has a rich history that spans thousands of years and encompasses various styles and traditions.

Historical records suggest that Qigong originated in ancient China, with some references dating back over 5,000 years. It draws upon traditional Chinese medicine, Taoist philosophy, and martial arts principles. Initially developed as a way to promote health and longevity, Qigong later incorporated spiritual and meditative aspects.

Qigong encompasses exercises and practices, including gentle movements, standing or seated postures, breathing techniques, and mental focus. These exercises aim to enhance the flow of Qi, harmonize the body's energy systems, and cultivate a state of balance and well-being. Some Qigong styles also incorporate visualization, sound, and self-massage techniques.

The benefits of practicing Qigong are multifaceted and can be experienced on physical, mental, and energetic levels. Here are some potential benefits:

Enhancing Energy and Vitality: Qigong aims to cultivate and harmonize the body's Qi, promoting a free energy flow throughout the body. This can lead to increased vitality, improved stamina, and overall well-being.

Stress Reduction and Relaxation: Qigong incorporates slow, gentle movements, deep breathing techniques, and focused attention, which can induce relaxation, reduce stress, and improve mental clarity.

Improving Physical Health: Regular Qigong practice can improve balance, flexibility, coordination, and posture. It may also strengthen muscles, tendons, and ligaments, promoting physical health and reducing the risk of injuries.

Supporting Emotional Well-being: Qigong's emphasis on mindfulness and deep breathing can help calm the mind, reduce anxiety, and improve emotional stability. It is believed to enhance self-awareness and promote a sense of inner peace.

Boosting Immune Function: Some studies suggest that Qigong practice can positively affect the immune system, potentially enhancing immune function and increasing the body's resistance to illness and disease.

Enhancing Mental Focus and Clarity: The meditative aspects of Qigong can help improve concentration, mental clarity, and focus. It may also contribute to better cognitive function and memory.

Promoting a Holistic Approach to Health: Qigong emphasizes the connection between the mind, body, and spirit. Harmonizing these aspects aims to promote overall health and well-being on multiple levels.

Tai Chi

Another ancient movement practice is Tai Chi. Tai Chi, also known as Tai Chi Chuan, is a traditional Chinese martial art that has evolved into a popular exercise and mindfulness practice. Its origins can be traced back to ancient China, with its development primarily attributed to Zhang Sanfeng, a legendary Taoist monk, in the 12th century.

Historically, Tai Chi was practiced as a martial art and self-defense system. Its movements are inspired by the principles of Yin and Yang, incorporating slow, flowing movements that emphasize balance, harmony, and internal energy cultivation. Over time, Tai Chi also became recognized for its health benefits and began to be practiced for therapeutic purposes.

Tai Chi gained widespread popularity in the 20th century when it was promoted as a form of exercise that could benefit both physical and mental well-being. The Chinese government significantly promoted Tai Chi by standardizing and popularizing various forms and creating simplified routines suitable for a wide range of individuals.

Today, Tai Chi is practiced worldwide for its numerous health benefits. It is commonly recommended for individuals of all ages and fitness levels due to its gentle and low-impact nature. Some of the recognized health benefits of Tai Chi include:

Improved balance and flexibility: Tai Chi incorporates slow and controlled movements, promoting better balance, coordination, and flexibility. This can be especially beneficial for older adults in reducing the risk of falls and improving overall physical function.

Stress reduction and relaxation: The mindful and meditative aspects of Tai Chi help promote relaxation, reduce stress, and improve mental well-being. Focused breathing and slow movements can have a calming effect on the mind and body.

Strength and muscle tone: Despite its gentle nature, Tai Chi can help improve muscle strength and tone, particularly in the lower body. The controlled movements engage various muscle groups, contributing to overall strength and endurance.

Cardiovascular health: Although less intense than traditional cardiovascular exercises, practicing Tai Chi has improved cardiovascular fitness, including lower blood pressure, reduced heart rate, and enhanced circulation.

Mental clarity and cognitive function: Regular practice of Tai Chi has been linked to improved cognitive function, including enhanced concentration, memory, and mental clarity. It may also positively impact anxiety, depression, and sleep quality.

Overall well-being: Tai Chi promotes a holistic approach to health, addressing physical and mental aspects. Its gentle movements and focus on internal energy flow are believed to harmonize the body and mind, promoting overall well-being.

Greek Gymnastics

Greek gymnastics, known as "gymnastikē" in ancient Greece, held a significant place in Greek society and culture. The history of Greek gymnastics can be traced back to as early as the 7th century BCE and continued to flourish until the decline of the Greek civilization.

History: Gymnastics in ancient Greece was closely associated with education, military training, and pursuing physical excellence. It was an integral part of the Greek educational system, particularly for young males, and aimed to develop a well-rounded individual with physical strength, agility, and mental discipline.

The ancient Greeks considered the human body as an expression of beauty, strength, and grace, emphasizing the cultivation of the body through physical exercises and activities. Gymnastics was not only seen as a means to enhance physical fitness but also as a way to cultivate moral virtues, discipline, and a strong character.

Benefits: The practice of Greek gymnastics offered numerous benefits, both physical and mental. Some of the key benefits associated with Greek gymnastics in ancient times include:

Physical Fitness: Greek gymnastics helped develop physical strength, flexibility, endurance, and overall fitness. Various exercises and activities such as running, jumping, wrestling, discus throwing, and calisthenics were employed to improve muscle tone, coordination, and overall physical prowess.

Military Training: Gymnastics played a crucial role in preparing young men for military service. It developed essential skills such as agility, balance, hand-eye coordination, and the ability to endure physically demanding tasks on the battlefield.

Character Development: Greek gymnastics was seen as a means of instilling discipline, self-control, and moral virtues in individuals. It fostered qualities such as perseverance, courage, teamwork, and the pursuit of excellence.

Mental Focus and Clarity: The rigorous physical training and disciplined approach to gymnastics in ancient Greece were believed to enhance mental focus, concentration, and clarity. It promoted mental toughness and the ability to overcome challenges.

Social Integration: Gymnastics was often practiced in communal settings such as gymnasiums, where individuals came together to train and compete. This provided opportunities for social interactions, camaraderie, and the developing of a sense of community.

Aesthetic Appreciation: Greek gymnastics celebrated the beauty of the human body and emphasized the harmony of movement and form. It fostered an appreciation for physical aesthetics and the integration of grace and strength.

Overall Well-being: Greek gymnastics aimed to cultivate a balanced and harmonious individual by addressing both physical and mental aspects of well-being. It promoted a holistic approach to health, recognizing the interconnection between the body, mind, and spirit.

It's important to note that our understanding of Greek gymnastics is derived from historical writings, artistic depictions, and archaeological evidence. The ancient Greek approach to gymnastics was distinct from modern gymnastics, encompassing a broader range of physical activities and deeply embedded in their culture and societal values.

While ancient Greek gymnastics no longer exists in its original form, its legacy has influenced the development of modern sports and physical education practices.

Martial Arts

The history of Chinese martial arts, also known as Wushu or Kung Fu, is rich and spans thousands of years. Chinese martial arts originated in ancient China and evolved as a combination of self-defense techniques, physical training, philosophy, and traditional Chinese medicine.

History: Chinese martial arts can be traced back to ancient China, with roots in the legendary Yellow Emperor Huangdi and the Xia Dynasty (circa 2205-1766 BCE). Various factors, including warfare, hunting techniques, cultural exchange, and the philosophies of Taoism, Buddhism, and Confucianism, influenced Chinese martial arts development.

Over centuries, Chinese martial arts systems developed and diversified, with different styles emerging in different regions of China. These styles were often associated with famous martial artists, legendary figures, or specific monastic traditions.

Benefits: Chinese martial arts offer a wide range of benefits, encompassing physical, mental, and spiritual aspects. Some of the key benefits associated with the practice of Chinese martial arts include:

Self-Defense: Chinese martial arts emphasize practical self-defense techniques and strategies, equipping practitioners with the skills and confidence to protect themselves if necessary.

Physical Fitness: Martial arts training involves rigorous physical exercises, such as stances, kicks, punches, and forms (katas). Regular practice can improve strength, flexibility, endurance, coordination, balance, and overall physical fitness.

Discipline and Focus: Martial arts training instills discipline, focus, and mental concentration. The demanding nature of practice requires practitioners to concentrate on their movements, leading to improved mental clarity and focus in other aspects of life.

Character Development: Chinese martial arts aim to cultivate positive character traits and virtues, such as respect, humility, perseverance, patience, and self-control. Practitioners are encouraged to embody these qualities in training and daily life.

Stress Reduction and Mental Well-being: Martial arts practice provides a channel for stress release and promotes mental well-being. Combining physical exercise, breath control, and meditative aspects can help reduce stress, enhance relaxation, and improve emotional balance.

Cultural Preservation and Appreciation: Chinese martial arts are deeply rooted in Chinese culture and heritage. Practicing martial arts allows individuals to connect with and preserve this cultural legacy, promoting a sense of identity, history, and tradition.

Spiritual Growth: Some Chinese martial arts systems incorporate philosophical and spiritual aspects, drawing from Taoism, Buddhism, or other belief systems. The practice of martial arts can serve as a path for personal growth, self-discovery, and the cultivation of inner harmony.

Community and Social Connections: Martial arts training often occurs in group settings, fostering a sense of community, camaraderie, and mutual support among practitioners. It provides opportunities for social connections and cultural exchange.

It's important to note that the benefits of Chinese martial arts can vary depending on the style, training methods, and individual practice. To fully experience the benefits, it is advisable to learn from qualified instructors who can guide practitioners in proper techniques, provide a supportive learning environment, and impart the underlying philosophy and principles of the specific martial art style.

Tribal Dance

Tribal dances have a long and diverse history, as they have been a significant part of cultural traditions in various indigenous communities worldwide. These dances hold deep cultural, spiritual, and social significance for the tribes, often passed down from generation to generation. Here, we will discuss the general history and potential benefits of tribal dance.

History: The history of tribal dance is deeply intertwined with indigenous peoples' histories, traditions, and customs. These dances have been performed for various reasons, such as celebrating important events, religious ceremonies, rites of passage, storytelling, community bonding, and expressing cultural identity.

Tribal dances have been practiced by indigenous communities worldwide, including Native American tribes, African tribes, Aboriginal tribes in Australia, Maori tribes in New Zealand, and many others. Each tribe has unique dance forms, movements, rhythms, and costumes, reflecting their cultural heritage and beliefs.

Benefits: Tribal dance offers numerous benefits, both to individuals and the community as a whole. Some potential benefits include:

Cultural Preservation: Tribal dance is crucial in preserving and passing down cultural traditions, stories, values, and ancestral knowledge from one generation to the next. It helps maintain a sense of identity, heritage, and continuity within indigenous communities.

Community Cohesion: Tribal dances are often performed in community settings, promoting a sense of togetherness, unity, and social cohesion. They provide opportunities for community members to come together, celebrate, and strengthen their bonds.

Physical Fitness: Tribal dances are typically energetic and require physical movement, contributing to improved fitness, flexibility, coordination, and overall well-being. Regular practice can enhance stamina, strength, and body awareness.

Emotional Expression: Tribal dance allows individuals to express their emotions, feelings, and experiences through movement and rhythm. It provides a creative outlet for self-expression, personal storytelling, and emotional release.

Spiritual Connection: Many tribal dances have deep spiritual significance, connecting dancers with their ancestors, the natural world, and the divine. These dances are often performed as part of religious or ceremonial practices, fostering a sense of spirituality and connection to the sacred.

Mind-Body Connection: Tribal dances often involve synchronized movements with music, enhancing the mind-body connection. This movement, rhythm, and breath integration can promote mindfulness, focus, and a heightened sense of present-moment awareness.

Well-being and Joy: Participating in tribal dances can bring joy, happiness, and fulfillment. The rhythmic movements, music, and communal atmosphere can uplift spirits, reduce stress, and improve overall mental and emotional well-being.

Cultural Exchange and Appreciation: Tribal dances provide cultural exchange and understanding opportunities between communities. Sharing dances with others promotes mutual respect, appreciation for diversity, and the preservation of indigenous cultures on a broader scale.

It's essential to recognize that tribal dances are deeply rooted in specific cultural contexts, and each tribe's dances hold unique meanings and significance. To truly understand the history, benefits, and nuances of tribal dance, it is essential to engage with and learn from the communities themselves, respecting their cultural protocols and seeking guidance from tribal members or cultural authorities.

This is by no means a complete list. It gives you an idea of the depth and breadth of movement practices available. You might create your own!

From Acrobatics to Zumba, for everyone, there is a movement style that will resonate. Finding that movement and incorporating it into your life will be transformational. Find it, and become who you really are.

Try it; you'll like it!

What moves you may be different at various times in your life. Trying other things helps you understand each practice's benefits on your unique constitution. In the You Playbook section, you'll see some suggestions. Try them for at least a couple of weeks before you decide which ones work best for you.

Chapter 9

What are you eating, and what is it doing?

I want to start talking about food. It's part of the intake that we're going to discuss. This is a HUGE subject, and I will probably go on and on. I've decided to take some of the information you might not be interested in and put it as an additional chapter at the back. I'll call this chapter "extras".

The reason for this is the way your food is grown, i.e., conventionally, organically, or regeneratively, matters a lot. For some of you, the term regenerative agriculture might be brand new, so I'll fill you in on that in the extras chapter.

For the record, when I say grown, I also include how animal products are produced.

For me, understanding how we produce our food is essential. If it isn't something you want to delve into, then I will ask you to take my word for it that how your food is grown has a MASSIVE impact on the nutritional value and levels of phytonutrients. I will explain shortly why phytonutrients matter so much in a later section. In order of nutritional value, here is how I rank food value:

1. Home-grown or locally grown using regenerative growing methods.
2. Homegrown or locally grown using organic methods
3. Regionally grown organically or regeneratively by farms where you can verify their methods.
4. Regeneratively grown anywhere
5. Organically grown anywhere
6. Non-certified organically grown but transitioning into organically grown anywhere
7. Conventionally grown using practices that minimize chemical use. This can be greenhouse-grown or a smaller farm that uses fewer chemicals.
8. Conventionally grown, monocropped

Finding the highest quality food is really important. https://www.frontiersin.org/articles/10.3389/fsufs.2021.699147/full is a good article if you want to go deeper. How food is grown matters to the levels of nutrients and phytochemicals. Conventionally grown will have the lowest nutritional value.

Phytos are Fantastic!

A phytonutrient is a natural compound that contributes to the plant's health, usually by protecting it from pests, UV rays, or disease. When humans eat plants, these phytonutrients can also provide health benefits. They're like nature's medicine, helping our bodies fight diseases and stay healthy.

There are tens of thousands of phytonutrients in the plant world. Many of these haven't been explored by the scientific community at all. These phytonutrients do amazing things in your body.

We're about to go into a semi-deep dive into food and how it is grown. It matters a lot, but I understand if you don't want

YOUR REAL BMI ~ 75

to go all the way into the dive with me. Here is what is critical for you to know:

PHYTONUTRIENTS CAN CHANGE YOUR LIFE!!

Phytonutrients, or phytos as we'll refer to them from now on, are plant compounds that help your body to experience wildly resilient good health. They are naturally occurring compounds in foods, and they perform different functions in the body.

Phytos are the foundation of Herbalism. They are part of the ancient wisdom passed down for millennia. When you hear "Eat the rainbow," think of those colors as having different magical powers. Not just one magical power, but many, many magical powers packed in every bite.

A diversity of phytos is the key to strong energy, immune function, healthy aging, and all aspects of your wellness. They can calm you down or help clear toxins. They can energize you. They can support vital functions. Plants and humans are meant to be together a lot more than we currently are.

Plants have so many ways to make you healthier. Phytos can perform miracles in the body, most of which haven't been well studied. As they say, there is no broccoli lobby, and unless there is a profit to be made, plant studies don't get well funded except if they might yield a pharmaceutical that can be patented.

By having a wide diversity of phytos in your body, you are giving yourself a farmacy of exciting compounds that are working for you without any effort on your part besides eating them.

Phytos can be system or organ-specific. They can be tropho-restorative, meaning they have a healing or restorative action on an organ or tissue.

Herbalism is commonly called plant medicine because of plants' efficacy in driving human health. You don't have to learn Herbalism (although it's a great field of study) to reap the benefits. You simply need to include diverse, fresh foods in your intake.

It can be as simple as adding fresh herbs to your cooking. Maybe put something different in your salad daily that you don't usually eat. Adding these things can give you so many benefits.

Many pharmaceuticals come from plants. Aspirin came from White Willow bark. The difference between the two is that when you take White Willow bark, there are a host of synergies that the plant has that the aspirin does not.

Meats raised correctly also contain plant phytos, so don't think this is a vegetarianism lecture. Animals intuitively eat certain plants, and when they have access to them, they consume wide varieties. My chickens love to grab greens from the garden and eat a lot of weeds.

The point that I want to drive home is that eating with phytos in mind will change everything.

The one thing you can change now, regardless of how you're eating, is to increase the diversity of your food choices.

Adding diversity gives you more phytos. Phytos are superheroes working for you night and day. Get as many of them as you can.

Now for a deeper dive if you're interested:

Let's explore some of the known phytos. When you read this, remember that there are *tens of thousands* of these phytos:

Lycopene:

- Found in: Tomatoes, watermelons, pink grapefruits, and guavas.
- Benefits: Lycopene is a powerful antioxidant linked to reduced risk of certain cancers, especially prostate cancer.

It also promotes heart health and may protect against sunburn.

- Curcumin:
  - Found in: Turmeric.
  - Benefits: Curcumin is renowned for its potent anti-inflammatory and antioxidant properties. It's been studied for its roles in fighting cancer, treating depressive disorders, and reducing the risk of heart disease.
- Quercetin:
  - Found in: Onions, apples, berries, and many other fruits and vegetables.
  - Benefits: Quercetin possesses anti-inflammatory, antihistamine, and antioxidant properties. It may help alleviate allergies, lower blood pressure, and reduce the risk of chronic diseases.
- Anthocyanins:
  - Found in: Blueberries, cherries, blackberries, raspberries, red cabbage, and red grapes. It is also found in Elderberry, a powerful antiviral
  - Benefits: These powerful antioxidants may protect cells from damage, lower blood pressure, reduce inflammation, and decrease the risk of heart disease and certain cancers.
- Resveratrol:
  - Found in: Red wine, red grapes, peanuts, and some berries.
  - Benefits: Resveratrol has antioxidant and anti-inflammatory effects. It's been studied for its potential to increase lifespan, protect against heart disease, and inhibit the spread of cancer cells.
- Glucosinolates:
  - Found in: Cruciferous vegetables like broccoli, Brussels sprouts, cabbage, and kale.

- Benefits: When these compounds are broken down (like during chewing or chopping), they form other compounds that have been shown to inhibit the growth of cancer cells.
- Epigallocatechin gallate (EGCG):
  - Found in: Green tea.
  - Benefits: EGCG is a potent antioxidant that may protect against heart disease, reduce the risk of certain cancers, and support brain health.
- Saponins:
  - Found in: Beans, chickpeas, and quinoa.
  - Benefits: Saponins have antioxidant, immune-boosting, and cholesterol-lowering properties.
- Allicin:
  - Found in: Garlic and onions.
  - Benefits: Allicin has antimicrobial properties and may help reduce blood pressure and cholesterol levels.
- Lutein and Zeaxanthin:
- Found in: Spinach, kale, corn, eggs, and other vegetables.
- Benefits: These carotenoids are vital for eye health. They protect against damaging light and may reduce the risk of age-related macular degeneration.

We don't have good data on how the various man-made chemicals interact in human bodies. We also don't have good data on how the various phytos interact in the human body,

What we do know indicates that these phytos are protective and rejuvenating and can have a profoundly positive effect on all metrics of our well-being. We know that they interact synergistically to increase health.

Don't we want a lot more of these in our bodies? Imagine your body having the tools to fix things before you know something is off. By eating correctly, we are filling our body with this fantastic toolbox that does things to keep us healthy, happy, and more energetic. And we don't have to do a thing except make the food choices that support this!

If I am what I eat, do I know what I'm eating?

I've hosted many visitors from around the globe, and they all speak about how different the U.S. food system is. Many additives and other substances banned from foods in the E.U. and other places across the globe are allowed in the U.S. food system.

The way your food is grown matters a lot. The amount of phytonutrients in food can differ significantly based on how it is grown. How can you get the most phytonutrient-rich food?

There are some excellent strategies to adopt no matter where you are:

1. **Can you grow some food yourself?** Even a pot on the counter with an array of herbs growing can begin to make a difference. If you don't want to plant a garden, are there people in your area who will plant and maintain one for you in your yard?
2. **Volunteer in a garden.** There are over *forty thousand* gardens in the U.S. that are growing food for food banks. Volunteering at one teaches you a lot and exposes you to some great soil organisms that will help you be healthier.
3. **Join a CSA.** CSA stands for community-supported agriculture. It's you interacting directly with the farmer and getting a weekly harvest share during your growing season. This means you're eating the food within a week or so of harvest, which is important.
4. **Find local growers** and ask them what farmers' markets or local stores they supply. Ask them what day they deliver and shop on that day.

5. **Learn to forage** and eat the weeds! In my yard, I have many yummy edible weeds that I eat. My soil is excellent, and my daily salad has some great phytos.
6. **Learn about the importance of soil quality** and find food being produced regeneratively. You'll learn more about the term "regenerative" and how it applies to food quality in the "extras" chapter.

FUN FACT: Did you know that free-range meat contains phytos, but industrialized meat does not? The animals eat various plants, and you also benefit from their varied diets. If meat is in your diet, make it free-range whenever possible.

Buying organic is important not just because of the absence of chemicals. Organic methods, especially regenerative methods, will increase the concentration and diversity of phytos in your food.

Buying organic produce can be more expensive, but as more of us choose organic or refuse to buy foods that don't have good growing practices, we can make access to real food more common. The other thing about buying good, whole foods is that you get a lot more nutrition in the calories you consume. For many people, this results in a marked decrease in the volume of food they eat. Well-nourished people have less deficit-driven cravings.

Another area that you might enjoy but can skip if you don't:

Let's get into a little bit about the importance of growing techniques. Conventional farming relies heavily on inputs like chemical fertilizers and pesticides to manage large fields of the same crop stretching as far as the eye can see.

Regenerative farming relies heavily on systems that have been proven to be effective since nature began feeding us. To understand regenerative farming, we must understand using inputs versus working with a closed-loop system.

A closed-loop system is precisely what it sounds like. Nothing comes in, and everything is reused or recycled. Nature is a closed-loop system. Trees drop their leaves, and insects and bacteria break the nutrients from them down to be recycled and reused. It is the same with everything in nature.

The way I like to put it is that one thing's poop is another thing's pudding. The natural cycle means that there is no waste. It also does many other things for the planet and the beings that live on it. A closed-loop system means that everything in the system is provided for, and the earth stays in balance.

Our current agricultural system relies heavily on inputs. Think of it as being like an infant. An input-reliant system relies on outside forces to meet all its needs like an infant. Recently, fertilizer prices spiked, and some farms returned to using manures. This was good for the soil because it fed soil bacteria.

Inputs are things that are added. In regenerative gardening, we use natural inputs such as manures, tree mulch, eggshells, etc. Conventional gardening/farming inputs are usually chemicals, like chemical fertilizers. When we use chemical inputs, we disrupt the natural cycle in many ways.

Extracting the components for inorganic fertilizers destroys habitats and contaminates ecosystems. Chemical fertilizers don't provide the bacteria and other soil web components with the nutrition they need to survive. Dead soil webs mean inefficient use of inputs by the plants, requiring more inputs, resulting in runoffs and dead zones.

We took a perfect system and broke it down into parts. We then assumed we understood the parts and proceeded to re-arrange them. It's been a total ecological disaster that we can reverse with regenerative farming methods.

What we missed completely by embracing modern farming techniques is that growing food isn't just about the food. It is about the system. The soil web is the true magic in the regenerative nature of our world. To fully appreciate the difference between mono-cropped and regeneratively grown food, it is essential to understand the soil web.

The soil web is crucial in supporting plant growth and overall soil health. Here's a simplified explanation of how it works:

Nutrient Cycling: The organisms in the soil web break down organic matter, such as decaying plant material or animal waste, into smaller components. They release nutrients in forms that plants can absorb and use for their growth and development. This process is known as nutrient cycling.

Soil Structure: The activities of soil organisms, particularly earthworms and burrowing insects, help to create tunnels and spaces in the soil. These tunnels improve soil structure, allowing water to infiltrate more easily and roots to grow deeper, leading to healthier and more resilient plants.

Disease Suppression: Certain beneficial microorganisms, such as mycorrhizal fungi, can form a symbiotic relationship with plant roots. They help plants absorb nutrients more efficiently and protect against harmful pathogens by competing for resources or releasing compounds that inhibit their growth.

Decomposition and Organic Matter Breakdown: Soil organisms like bacteria and fungi are crucial in breaking down organic matter, such as fallen leaves or dead plant material. This decomposition process releases nutrients into the soil, enriching it and supporting future plant growth.

When food is grown in soil with a healthy and diverse soil web, several positive outcomes can be observed:

Nutrient-rich foods: The nutrient cycling facilitated by the soil web helps plants access a wide range of essential nutrients, resulting in more nutrient-rich crops.

Enhanced Flavor and Aroma: Healthy soil ecosystems can improve food taste, flavor, and aroma profiles. This is partly due to diverse soil microorganisms interacting with plant roots and influencing the production of certain compounds responsible for sensory attributes.

Resilient Plants: The presence of beneficial microorganisms and well-structured soil can make plants more resilient to stress, such as drought or disease, resulting in healthier and higher-quality crops.

In contrast, when food is grown in soils lacking a robust soil web, several adverse outcomes may occur:

Nutrient Depletion: With a diverse soil web, the nutrient cycling process may be protected, reducing nutrient availability for plants and potentially resulting in nutrient-deficient crops.

Increased Disease Susceptibility: Without beneficial microorganisms that suppress disease, plants may become more susceptible to harmful pathogens, increasing the risk of plant diseases.

Soil Degradation: Soils lacking a healthy soil web can experience reduced organic matter content, poor soil structure, and erosion, leading to soil degradation and decreased fertility.

The depletion of our soil and the destruction of the soil web have created terrible consequences for our food system. Nature had a perfect system. We thought we could do better. We can't.

If you take it a few steps further, it is intuitive to understand that nature's perfect system includes perfection for human bodies. We evolved in harmony with soil bacteria.

Bacteria protect our skin, digest our food, and so much more. When you do the numbers, you are only 10% human; the rest are beneficial bacteria. Interacting with the bacteria in the natural world is how we acquire and replenish our bacteria.

You might have been delivered via C-section if born in the developed world. Since the trip down the birth control is vital to creating a healthy microbiome, this is a problem. The time in the birth canal serves to give the infant its first serving of healthy bacteria.

Today, it is known that packing the mother's vagina with gauze and wiping the baby with that gauze helps mitigate the loss of time in the birth canal for c-section babies. We've demonized bacteria for a long time without understanding their vital role in human health.

When you realize that the studies in human health and bacteria, especially gut bacteria, became prominent in the 90s, you wonder how much else we don't know about human health and how we interact with the natural world. If we didn't understand the importance of gut bacteria until relatively recently, what else are we missing?

Chapter 10

Magic in my kitchen

The real problem with eating many processed foods or a diet heavy on meat products is that you are missing the opportunities to ingest all these amazing phytos!

Let's look at some common kitchen herbs to give a small snapshot of how ingesting plants can make a huge difference in human health.

There are as many examples of the healing properties of plants as there are plants. We will look at a few common herbs to give us a small glimpse into what plants can do for us.

I chose these four herbs because they have been commonly used for so long that there is even a folk song about them. I just want to drive home that there is magic in whole, plant-based foods. You can skip this if you're already convinced.

Parsley (Petroselinum crispum) is a popular herb widely used in culinary preparations worldwide. It is native to the Mediterranean region and belongs to the Apiaceae family. Parsley is a flavorful herb and a good source of various nutrients. Let's explore the chemical constituents of parsley and its potential health benefits:

Essential oils: Parsley contains essential oils such as myristicin, limonene, eugenol, and alpha-thujene. These oils contribute to the herb's aromatic properties and have anti-oxidant, antimicrobial, and anti-inflammatory effects.

Flavonoids: Parsley is rich in flavonoids, including apigenin, luteolin, and kaempferol. Flavonoids are known for their anti-oxidant and anti-inflammatory properties, and they may help protect against chronic diseases and support overall health.

Vitamins and minerals: Parsley is a nutrient-dense herb that provides various vitamins and minerals. It is exceptionally high in vitamins K, C, A, and folate. It also contains smaller amounts of other minerals like potassium, calcium, and iron.

Now, let's explore some of the health benefits associated with parsley:

Antioxidant effects: The flavonoids and essential oils in parsley have antioxidant properties that help protect cells from damage caused by free radicals. Antioxidants reduce the risk of chronic diseases, including heart disease, cancer, and neurodegenerative disorders.

Anti-inflammatory properties: The flavonoids and essen-tial oils in parsley help reduce inflammation. Chronic inflam-mation is linked to various diseases, such as arthritis, heart disease, and certain cancers. Including parsley in your diet can contribute to an overall anti-inflammatory effect.

Digestive health: Parsley has been traditionally used as a digestive aid. It can help stimulate digestion, promote healthy bowel movements, and alleviate bloating and flatulence. The essential oils in parsley also have antimicrobial properties that can help combat harmful bacteria in the gut.

Bone health: Parsley is a rich source of vitamin K, which plays a vital role in bone health and blood clotting. Adequate vitamin K intake is associated with improved bone density and reduced risk of fractures. Including parsley in your diet can help support strong and healthy bones.

Immune support: Parsley contains vitamin C, essential for a healthy immune system. Vitamin C helps stimulate the production of white blood cells, which fight off infections and support overall immune function.

Diuretic properties: Parsley has diuretic properties, meaning it may help increase urine production and promote the elimination of waste products from the body. This can be beneficial for individuals with fluid retention or urinary tract issues.

Fresh breath: Parsley is often used as a natural breath freshener. Its high chlorophyll content helps neutralize odors and freshens breath.

It's worth noting that while parsley is generally safe when consumed in culinary amounts, concentrated parsley extracts or supplements should be used with caution, especially in large doses. As with any herbal remedy, it's advisable to consult a healthcare professional before using parsley for medicinal purposes, especially if you have any underlying health conditions or are taking medications.

Sage (Salvia officinalis) is an aromatic herb used for centuries for its culinary and medicinal properties. It is native to the Mediterranean region and belongs to the Lamiaceae family. Sage is known for its distinctive flavor, fragrance, and potential health benefits. Let's explore the chemical constituents of sage and its health benefits:

Essential oils: Sage contains essential oils, including thujone, cineole, camphor, and borneol. These oils contribute to the herb's aroma and may have antimicrobial, anti-inflammatory, and antioxidant properties.

Flavonoids: Sage is rich in flavonoids such as apigenin, luteolin, and rosmarinic acid. Flavonoids are known for their antioxidant and anti-inflammatory effects and can reduce the risk of chronic diseases

Rosmarinic acid: This compound is found in sage and is known for its antioxidant and anti-inflammatory properties.

Rosmarinic acid can help protect cells from damage caused by free radicals and reduce inflammation in the body.

Now, let's explore some health benefits associated with sage:

Cognitive health: Sage has traditionally been used to support cognitive function and memory. Some research suggests that sage extract may improve cognitive performance and memory in healthy individuals and those with mild cognitive impairment. The compounds in sage may positively impact brain function and protect against neurodegenerative diseases.

Antimicrobial properties: The essential oils in sage, such as thujone and camphor, possess antimicrobial properties. They may help inhibit the growth of bacteria, viruses, and fungi, making sage beneficial for oral health and respiratory conditions.

Anti-inflammatory effects: Sage contains compounds, including rosmarinic acid, with anti-inflammatory properties. These compounds help reduce inflammation, benefiting conditions like arthritis and inflammatory bowel diseases.

Digestive health: Sage has been traditionally used to support digestion. It may help stimulate the production of digestive enzymes, alleviate bloating and flatulence, and aid in the digestion of fats. Sage tea or infusions may be consumed for these digestive benefits.

Antioxidant activity: Sage contains various compounds with antioxidant properties, such as flavonoids and rosmarinic acid. Antioxidants help neutralize harmful free radicals in the body and protect cells from oxidative stress. This may reduce the risk of chronic diseases, including certain cancers and cardiovascular disorders.

Oral health: The antimicrobial properties of sage may be beneficial for oral health. Sage mouthwashes or rinses may help reduce plaque formation, gingivitis, and bad breath. Sage-infused products are commonly used in natural oral care.

Menopausal symptoms: Sage has been traditionally used to alleviate menopausal symptoms like hot flashes and night sweats. Some studies suggest that sage extract may help reduce the frequency and intensity of these symptoms, although further research is needed to confirm its effectiveness.

As with any herbal remedy, it's essential to consult a healthcare professional before using sage for medicinal purposes, especially if you have any underlying health conditions or are taking medications. Additionally, using sage in culinary amounts or as directed by a qualified practitioner is advisable, as concentrated forms or high doses may have potential side effects.

Rosemary (Rosmarinus officinalis) is a famous culinary and medicinal herb native to the Mediterranean region. It has been used for centuries for its aromatic properties and potential health benefits. Rosemary contains a variety of chemical constituents that contribute to its therapeutic properties. Here are some of the critical constituents found in rosemary:

Rosmarinic acid: This compound is known for its antioxidant and anti-inflammatory properties. It helps protect cells from damage caused by free radicals and may reduce inflammation.

Carnosic acid: Another potent antioxidant compound found in rosemary, carnosic acid, has been studied for its potential neuroprotective effects. It may help protect against neurodegenerative diseases like Alzheimer's and Parkinson's by reducing oxidative stress in the brain.

Essential oils: Rosemary contains volatile cineole, camphor, and alpha-pinene. These oils give rosemary its distinctive aroma and contribute to its antimicrobial, antifungal, and antiviral properties. They may also have a positive impact on respiratory health.

Flavonoids: Rosemary contains various flavonoids, including luteolin, apigenin, and diosmin. Flavonoids are known for their antioxidant and anti-inflammatory effects. They may help protect against chronic diseases like cancer and cardio-vascular disorders.

Now, let's explore some health benefits associated with rosemary:

Antioxidant properties: The antioxidants in rosemary, such as rosmarinic acid and carnosic acid, help combat oxidative stress and protect cells from damage. This may contribute to a reduced risk of chronic diseases, including certain types of cancer and cardiovascular disorders.

Anti-inflammatory effects: Rosemary has anti-inflamma-tory properties, which can benefit inflammation conditions like arthritis. Rosmarinic acid has been found to inhibit certain enzymes that promote inflammation in the body.

Cognitive health: Some studies suggest rosemary can positively affect memory, concentration, and overall cognitive function. The antioxidants and anti-inflammatory compounds in rosemary can help protect the brain from oxidative stress and inflammation, potentially reducing the risk of age-related cognitive decline.

Digestive health: Rosemary has traditionally been used to support digestion. It can help stimulate the production of digestive enzymes, improve bile flow, and alleviate symptoms such as indigestion, bloating, and flatulence.

Respiratory support: The essential oils in rosemary, particu-larly cineole, have expectorant properties and can help relieve respiratory conditions like coughs, bronchitis, and conges-tion. Inhalation of rosemary vapor or using rosemary-infused products may provide respiratory relief.

Hair and scalp health: Rosemary is commonly used in hair care products due to its benefits for the scalp and hair. It can promote hair growth, help combat dandruff, and improve the overall health and appearance of the hair.

Mood enhancement: The aroma of rosemary has been associated with improved mood, reduced stress, and increased alertness. Aromatherapy using rosemary essential oil can help uplift the mood and enhance mental clarity.

It's important to note that while rosemary has a long history of culinary and medicinal use, further scientific research is needed to fully understand its potential health benefits and determine optimal doses for specific conditions. Additionally, it's advisable to consult with a healthcare professional before using rosemary for medicinal purposes, especially if you have any underlying health conditions or are taking medications.

Thyme (Thymus vulgaris) is a perennial herb commonly used in culinary preparations and traditional medicine. It belongs to the Lamiaceae family and is native to the Mediterranean region. Thyme is known for its distinct aroma and flavor and offers potential health benefits. Let's explore the chemical constituents of thyme and its potential health benefits:

Essential oils: Thyme contains essential oils contributing to its characteristic aroma and flavor. The main components of thyme essential oil include thymol, carvacrol, p-cymene, and terpene. These oils possess antimicrobial, antifungal, and antioxidant properties.

Flavonoids: Thyme is rich in flavonoids, including luteolin, apigenin, and naringenin. Flavonoids are known for their antioxidant and anti-inflammatory effects, which may contribute to the potential health benefits of thyme.

Phenolic acids: Thyme contains various phenolic acids such as rosmarinic, caffeic, and ferulic. These compounds have antioxidant and anti-inflammatory properties and contribute to the overall health benefits of thyme.

Now, let's explore some of the health benefits of thyme:

Antimicrobial properties: Thyme essential oil, particularly its component thymol, exhibits potent antimicrobial activity against bacteria and fungi. It may help inhibit the growth of harmful microorganisms, making it helpful in preventing and treating various infections.

Antioxidant effects: Thyme is rich in antioxidants, including flavonoids and phenolic acids. These compounds help neutralize free radicals in the body, protecting cells from oxidative damage and potentially reducing the risk of chronic diseases such as cancer and cardiovascular disorders.

Respiratory health: Thyme has been traditionally used to support respiratory health. The essential oils in thyme, such as thymol and carvacrol, have expectorant properties and can help relieve coughs, congestion, and bronchitis. Thyme-infused steam inhalation or herbal teas can provide respiratory relief.

Digestive health: Thyme has been used to support digestion and alleviate digestive issues. It can help stimulate the production of digestive enzymes, improve digestion, and reduce symptoms such as bloating, gas, and indigestion.

Anti-inflammatory effects: Thyme flavonoids and phenolic acids have anti-inflammatory properties. These compounds may help reduce inflammation associated with various chronic diseases, including arthritis and inflammatory bowel diseases.

Immune support: Thyme contains compounds that can support immune function. The antimicrobial and antioxidant properties of thyme help strengthen the immune system and protect against infections.

Cognitive health: Some studies suggest thyme may have cognitive-enhancing effects. It may help improve memory, concentration, and overall cognitive function. The antioxidant and anti-inflammatory compounds in thyme contribute to its potential benefits for brain health.

It's important to note that while thyme is generally safe when used in culinary amounts, concentrated thyme extracts or supplements should be used with caution, especially in large doses. As with any herbal remedy, it's advisable to consult a healthcare professional before using thyme for medicinal

purposes, particularly if you have any underlying health conditions or are taking medications.

It is challenging to get data, but as of 2016, it was estimated
that 58% of the average American diet consisted of ultra-
processed foods. It's not just that most ultra-processed foods
are devoid of nutrients and full of sugar and other unhealthy
additives; it is also that in eating these, we are depriving our
diets of the foods that could help offset the damage of the
processed foods.

When you look at what these four simple herbs can do for
the human body, it's clear that nature has our backs, stomachs,
hearts, and everything else. These four herbs are not even
the tip of the iceberg regarding the fantastic world of plants.
By incorporating a diverse selection of plants into our diets,
we create an internal pharmacopeia to assist our bodies with
crucial functions.

*Rest and repair functions are most impaired when we have
micronutrient deficiencies, so it can take years or even dec-
ades for the full effect of our insufficient diets to create problems. In many cases, by the time we understand that we have
a problem, chronic disease, and sometimes deadly disease has
taken up residence in our bodies.*

In addition to micronutrient deficiencies, many of us aren't
getting enough fiber. Processed foods are usually fiber-poor;
supplemental fiber doesn't really solve that problem.

Fiber in food does many things. It can feed our gut bacteria,
leading to a healthier gut biome. A healthier gut biome supports overall bodily functions. Fiber helps slow sugar spikes,
helping us keep our insulin levels from spiking.

Our body signals to us what it needs. If your body is crying
out for fiber, there are likely other components in fiber-rich
food that your body needs. Natural foods have synergies. The
impact on your body is greater than the sum of the nutrients

inside the foods. Our bodies need whole foods for a multitude of reasons.

Taking a fiber supplement gives you one type of fiber, but fails to address the deficiencies in your gut. Your gut bacteria need to be fed. They are the ones doing the work in there!

Prebiotics is the word we use for the food that the probiotics eat. You want as much diversity as possible in your gut bacteria, and you do that by eating a diverse diet. Full stop. No shortcuts or supplements can fully make up for deficiencies in the gut.

Fiber is crucial in maintaining human health and essential to a balanced diet. It refers to the indigestible carbohydrates in plant foods, such as fruits, vegetables, whole grains, legumes, nuts, and seeds. Understanding fiber and its role in maintaining a healthy body is essential.

Digestive health: One of the primary benefits of fiber is its ability to promote healthy digestion. There are two types of fiber: soluble and insoluble. Soluble fiber dissolves in water, forming a gel-like substance in the digestive tract. Insoluble fiber, on the other hand, adds bulk to the stool. Both types contribute to regular bowel movements, preventing constipation and promoting overall digestive health. Fiber can also help prevent or alleviate conditions such as hemorrhoids, diverticulosis, and irritable bowel syndrome (IBS).

Weight management: High-fiber foods are generally less calorie-dense and more filling, aiding in weight management. Fiber adds bulk to the diet without contributing many calories, resulting in fullness and satisfaction. It can help control appetite, reduce overeating, and support healthy weight loss or maintenance. Additionally, high-fiber foods require more chewing, slowing the eating process and allowing the body to recognize satiety signals more effectively.

Blood sugar control: Fiber is significant in managing blood sugar levels, particularly for individuals with diabetes or insulin resistance. Soluble fiber slows down the digestion and absorption of carbohydrates, which leads to a gradual release of glucose into the bloodstream. This helps prevent spikes in blood sugar levels, promotes better glycemic control, and reduces the risk of developing type 2 diabetes. Including high-fiber foods in meals can also improve insulin sensitivity and contribute to overall metabolic health.

Heart health: A high-fiber diet has been associated with a reduced risk of heart disease. Soluble fiber helps lower LDL cholesterol (the "bad" cholesterol) by binding to bile acids, which are then excreted. This mechanism promotes the liver's use of cholesterol to produce more bile acids, decreasing circulating cholesterol levels. Fiber also supports a healthy cardiovascular system by reducing blood pressure, improving blood lipid profiles, and reducing inflammation.

Gut microbiome health: The gut microbiome refers to the diverse community of microorganisms in the digestive tract. Fiber acts as a prebiotic, providing nourishment to beneficial gut bacteria. These bacteria ferment the fiber, producing short-chain fatty acids (SCFAs) with numerous health benefits. SCFAs support the health of the intestinal cells, contribute to a healthy immune system, and help regulate inflammation in the gut. A diverse and balanced gut microbiome is crucial for overall health and has been linked to various aspects, including mental health and immune function.

Please note that it's recommended to increase fiber intake gradually and drink plenty of water alongside a high-fiber diet to prevent digestive discomfort. The recommended daily fiber intake varies depending on age, sex, and individual health needs, but most dietary guidelines suggest a target of around 25-30 grams per day for adults.

In summary, fiber plays a vital role in maintaining human health. It supports digestive health, aids in weight management, helps control blood sugar levels, promotes heart health, and contributes to a healthy gut microbiome. Including a variety of fiber-rich foods in the diet is crucial for reaping the benefits of fiber and maintaining overall well-being.

It's pretty intuitive if you think about it. You know how the food you eat makes you feel. Food isn't supposed to leave you bloated, lethargic, and tired. We shouldn't experience desperate cravings and mood swings from our food. Most importantly, food shouldn't contribute to premature aging, chronic disease, and early death. But processed food does all of these things.

There is a strong correlation between the rise in processed food consumption and the prevalence of lifestyle diseases such as diabetes, heart disease, and obesity.

These diseases have reached epidemic proportions in many countries, and dietary factors, including the increased consumption of processed foods, are believed to contribute to their development significantly.

Processed foods are typically high in added sugars, unhealthy fats, sodium, and refined carbohydrates while low in essential nutrients like fiber, vitamins, and minerals. This nutrient-poor, energy-dense composition can have several detrimental effects on health:

Obesity: Processed foods are often calorie-dense and palatable, making it easier to overconsume them. The excessive intake of processed foods, combined with sedentary lifestyles, can lead to energy imbalance and contribute to weight gain and obesity. Obesity is a significant risk factor for numerous lifestyle diseases, including diabetes, heart disease, and certain types of cancer.

Diabetes: The consumption of processed foods, particularly those high in added sugars and refined carbohydrates, has been strongly associated with an increased risk of type 2 diabetes. These foods cause rapid spikes in blood sugar levels, leading to insulin resistance over time. Insulin resistance is a key feature of type 2 diabetes, where the body's cells become less responsive to insulin, resulting in elevated blood sugar levels.

Heart Disease: Processed foods are often rich in unhealthy fats, including trans and saturated fats. These fats can raise low-density lipoprotein (LDL) cholesterol levels, often called "bad" cholesterol, and increase the risk of developing heart disease and cardiovascular complications. Additionally, the high sodium content in processed foods can contribute to high blood pressure, another risk factor for heart disease.

Inflammation and Chronic Diseases: Processed foods, especially those containing additives and preservatives, can promote chronic inflammation. Chronic inflammation is associated with various diseases, including heart disease, diabetes, certain types of cancer, and autoimmune conditions.

Nutrient Deficiencies: Processed foods are low in essential nutrients like fiber, vitamins, and minerals. A diet lacking in these nutrients can lead to deficiencies, impairing the body's ability to function optimally and increasing the risk of various diseases.

It is important to note that the impact of processed foods on health is not solely due to their nutrient composition. Processing methods, such as high-temperature cooking, can generate harmful substances like acrylamide or advanced glycation end products (AGEs), which are associated with an increased risk of certain diseases.

Experimentation is the way forward regarding food. Explore your area. Who is growing food within an hour of you, and how are they growing it? Can you find someone like me who might have free-range eggs, biodynamically grown fruits or veggies, or other things for sale that you can add to your food choices?

Learn foraging in your area. I forage in my yard because I've purposely allowed wild areas. Wild foods are deeply nutritious. When I'm eating a portion of wild food, I know that this plant out-competed the plants around it and grew with no help from anyone. It is likely full of strong phytos that will help my body.

Dollar weed is one of my favorite weeds. It tastes like water-cress and makes a lovely addition to a salad. Fresh herbs like oregano, tulsi, parsley, tarragon, and more mean that my salads are flavorful, and I can use just a bit of olive oil instead of an unhealthy processed dressing.

Temperate climates get some really wonderful spring weeds, like dandelion, burdock, stinging nettle, and more. Learning how to find and prepare these foods can add a lot of free nutrition to your life.

Chapter 11

Finding the
best food

WHY NOT GROW SOME FOOD?

We can look to history for some ideas. We currently mono-crop enough lawn grass in the U.S. to cover the state of Texas. That's estimated to be about 171 MILLION acres. What if we revived some strategies used to create Victory Gardens during WWII?

Victory gardens, also known as war gardens or food gardens for defense, are vegetable, fruit, and herb gardens cultivated by individuals and communities during war or food short-ages. Victory gardens gained prominence during World War I and World War II when nations faced significant challenges securing enough food for their populations and troops abroad. Here's some information about victory gardens:

Origin: The idea of victory gardens can be traced back to the early 19th century, but they became particularly popular during World War I and II. The term "victory garden" was coined in the United States during World War I, and the prac-tice was revived and expanded during World War II.

Purpose: Victory gardens were established to support the war effort and address food scarcity. By growing their food, individuals and communities could contribute to the overall food supply, allowing commercial agriculture to focus more on feeding soldiers and civilians abroad.

Scope: Victory gardens were not limited to private residences; schools, public parks, vacant lots, and other available spaces were also converted into productive gardens. The effort was collective, involving people of all ages and backgrounds.

Government Promotion: Governments played a significant role in promoting victory gardens. In the United States, the U.S. Department of Agriculture launched a national campaign called "War Food Administration" during World War II, encouraging citizens to grow their gardens. Posters, pamphlets, and media campaigns were used to spread the message.

Benefits: Victory Gardens had several advantages. They eased the food supply chain burden, reduced the strain on transportation systems, and helped ensure that troops had enough food to sustain themselves. Additionally, victory gardens were seen as morale boosters and contributed to a sense of patriotism and community spirit.

Legacy: Victory gardens had a lasting impact beyond the wars. They increased public awareness of agriculture and gardening, and many people continued gardening even after the wars ended. The concept of victory gardens has been revisited during economic hardship or crisis when access to food becomes a concern.

Modern Relevance: Though "victory gardens" are historically associated with wartime efforts, self-sufficiency, and community-based food production principles remain relevant today. Urban and community gardening has gained popularity in recent years as people seek to grow their food and promote sustainability.

By promoting self-reliance and community involvement, victory gardens played a significant role in helping nations weather the challenges of war and food shortages. They remain a symbol of resilience and unity during challenging times. Indeed, these are challenging times.

This is a call to action for all of us. It's an opportunity to strive for resilience in a time when climate change is likely to disrupt our food systems. Participating in some way in growing your food or supporting small, local food growers not only increases your resilience. Eating those foods will have a profound impact on your health.

When individuals transition from consuming processed foods to a diet consisting of whole, nutritious, and organically grown foods, they can experience several positive impacts on their bodies. Here are some key ways this dietary shift can affect the human body:

Nutrient Density: Whole, nutritious foods are rich in essential nutrients, including vitamins, minerals, fiber, and antioxidants. By incorporating these foods into their diet, individuals can ensure they are receiving a more comprehensive range of micronutrients necessary for optimal bodily functions, such as immune function, energy production, and cell repair.

Improved Digestive Health: Processed foods are often low in fiber, while whole foods are typically high in dietary fiber. Increasing fiber intake through entire foods aids digestion promotes regular bowel movements, and supports a healthy gut microbiome. This can reduce the risk of constipation, bloating, and other digestive issues.

Weight Management: Whole foods, particularly those in their natural state, are generally less calorie-dense than processed foods. They tend to be more satiating due to their higher fiber and protein content. Consequently, individuals may find it easier to control their calorie intake, maintain a healthy weight, and reduce the risk of obesity and associated conditions.

Enhanced Heart Health: A diet rich in whole, nutritious foods can contribute to better heart health. Whole foods are typically lower in unhealthy trans fats, added sugars, and sodium, which are prevalent in processed foods and have been linked to an increased risk of heart disease. Instead, whole foods provide heart-healthy nutrients such as omega-3 fatty acids, antioxidants, and fiber.

Reduced Inflammation: Processed foods often contain additives, artificial preservatives, and unhealthy fats that can promote inflammation. Conversely, whole foods, particularly those with anti-inflammatory properties, can help reduce chronic inflammation associated with various health issues, including cardiovascular disease, diabetes, and autoimmune conditions.

Balanced Blood Sugar Levels: Processed foods, especially those high in refined carbohydrates and added sugars, can cause rapid spikes in blood sugar levels. On the other hand, whole foods, particularly those with a lower glycemic index, release glucose more gradually, leading to more stable blood sugar levels. This can help prevent insulin resistance, type 2 diabetes, and metabolic syndrome.

Increased Energy and Vitality: Whole, nutrient-dense foods provide a steady energy supply due to their balanced macro-nutrient profile. By nourishing the body with high-quality nutrients, individuals may experience improved energy levels, reduced fatigue, and enhanced overall vitality.

Enhanced Skin Health: Nutrient-rich whole foods can contribute to healthier skin. Antioxidants found in fruits and vegetables help protect against oxidative stress, reducing the signs of aging and promoting a youthful complexion. Healthy fats from nuts, seeds, and avocados can also support skin hydration and suppleness.

Mental Well-being: While more research is needed, emerging evidence suggests a link between a healthy diet rich in whole foods and improved mental health. Nutrients such as omega-3 fatty acids, B vitamins, and antioxidants in whole foods may support brain function and reduce the risk of mental health disorders such as depression and anxiety.

It is worth noting that transitioning to a diet based on whole, nutritious foods requires a holistic approach considering individual preferences, dietary needs, and cultural factors.

In short, you are what you eat is more true than we might think. We all love those memes that say things like "Life is short; eat dessert first." "French fries are a vegetable," "Everything in moderation, including moderation."

While it is lovely to think that we can give in to the urge to see food as something we can eat strictly for enjoyment, it is not true. It is especially untrue in our world of toxicity and really bad food.

So, are we doomed? Do Twinkies win the day, and we all adjust to a life of medications, impairments, and feeling terrible most days? *NO!!!!!*

There is a learning curve and an adjustment to changing how we eat. It isn't always easy, but it will be one of the most rewarding and effective things you can do for Future You.

I see a lot of clients who tell me they are eating healthy. And they are eating well, based on the knowledge that they have. The key to this book, and why you're about to have an experience of food you've never had before, is that there is an easy way to understand how to eat to get the maximum benefit for your unique body.

Let me reiterate, in case you got lost in my rambles. If you skimmed through some parts, just be sure to read this:

The diversity of quality food you eat matters. You can add herbal teas, herbs, and spices to create some of that diversity. Your You Playbook will tell you what foods are great for you, but don't get caught up in finding favorites and thinking you can just eat those every day.

When making your changes, adding new foods is always easier than going down the deprivation path. If you have food addictions, removing those foods is the only answer. But if you don't have food addictions, you can gradually phase out the foods that aren't good for you as you slowly add more and more variety.

Change your food, and you change your life. Take the journey as an exciting adventure. Find a friend and take turns bringing a new food to the table or finding a new market. Make it fun!

Chapter 12

The Other Intake

The other Intake we'll discuss is everything else you allow in. Doom scrolling has become a widespread habit, and we're all falling for clickbait, especially when we think it will tell us what we want to hear.

From the movies we watch to the music we listen to, the people we hang out with, and the podcasters we follow, we allow other people access to our brains.

Our brains are supercomputers. When computers first became a thing, there was a common acronym: GIGO. It stood for garbage in, garbage out. It meant you'd have bad results if you put bad data or programming into the computer. Our brains are no different.

The most empowering thing you can do for your brain, emotional state, and mood is to control what goes in. Dr Andrew Huberman has a YouTube channel that can give you a deep dive into your neurochemistry.

The short version is that your brain does not know the difference between false and true information. It's just all information to your brain.

If you read and listen to continually negative news, your brain will think the world IS ending. You'll have the stress levels and other negative impacts of that subconscious belief, even if you don't consciously believe it.

If you listen to only positive news, your brain will think everything is good. Optimists live significantly longer than pessimists, so it's good for your health to be skewed toward the positive.

Since I know that negative news is everywhere, I consciously seek good news and positive vibes. Think about it like this: you have so many hours daily. The hours you might spend doom scrolling or listening to music that makes you sad or invokes bad memories does nothing for you.

On the other hand, music is a powerful motivator and mood enhancer. It's a fabulous tool. You can just keep it in the background, reminding your subconscious of your happiness.

Podcasts are great ways to engage with knowledge and keep up with the ever-changing world that we live in. You can expand your knowledge, and knowledge is power.

Creating a resilient mindset and holding mental boundaries gives you a silent partner in overall wellness.

Guided meditation, binaural beats, music, hypnosis, cognitive behavior therapy, and other mind modalities will help you reprogram your subconscious. A good exercise is to sit quietly and ask yourself: "What do I believe about myself and my future?"

If the answer isn't positive, then change it. Affirmations are great. I like to turn it into a song when I'm looking to create a thought pattern. Think of all the songs that get stuck in your head.

Wouldn't having a positive song stuck in your head be great? You can pick one you like, make up your own, or change the lyrics to a tune you love. I like to sing "Because I'm scrappy!" instead of "Because I'm happy!" to the Happy song by Pharell. It reminds me that I'm resilient and helps me feel strong when I need to overcome challenges.

At the same time, living in reality is important. If the house is on fire and you try to think it away, your brain will intercede and take the data from your sensory systems.

If you have real challenges, you have to face them. If you face a challenge feeling like you can't win, you're probably right. Thoughts like "I know this might be hard, but I can do it." "I'm strong enough to do this." "I got this!"

It's also good to make sure the people you go to for help are people that also believe in you.

You really are a temple. Treat yourself like one. Only allow things worthy of the awesomeness you are to enter into your body, mind, and field. You are in charge, and you've got this.

Chapter 13

THE FRAMEWORK

Now, let's get to the framework you will use to make choices in food, activities, and breathing techniques to support you.

This is the last piece of the puzzle you need to use your You Playbook.

In the back of this book, or the separate You Playbook, there is a system that will walk you through finding out which element(s) are dominant in your body and which are out of balance.

We've introduced the elements, and the You Playbook has information on each element. Let's dive into the framework!

In herbalism, we look at things through a particular lens. The elements play a big part. It's basically about where there might be an imbalance on the elemental spectrum. We call this the three polarities. The three polarities are an easy way to understand imbalances and propensities in people. These are the three polarities:

1. Hot-Cold,
2. Wet-Dry, and
3. Tense-Relaxed

If you listen to our language, you hear the elements used extensively to describe humans and human actions.

- "You should have seen him play. He was on fire!"
- "Don't ask her for help. She's cold."
- "John is such an airhead."
- "You need to ground that idea."
- "There she goes again, turning on the waterworks."

We unconsciously resonate with the natural system, and we often use the idea of the elements to describe what we are feeling or experiencing in our body.

The polarities are a simple way to understand using the elements to create balance and design your unique Secret Formula. This also gives you the tools to tweak your Secret Formula when things change.

What can make you need to change your Secret Formula?

- You move to another climate
- Life stress
- Illness
- Change of seasons
- You've corrected imbalances and don't need to adjust as much
- Any changing outside circumstance

Your Secret Formula is adaptive, making you more adaptive.

Back to the polarities. Here is a simple way to think about how you use the understanding of the polarities.

If it's hot, cool it down. This one is easy to recognize in things like fever and inflammation. We use a cool cloth (water) on someone's brow to cool a fever or a hot headache. We ice (water and ether) an injury to reduce inflammation.

If it's cold, warm it up. How often have you stamped your feet or rubbed your hands together to warm them? This increases circulation (fire) and warms you up. A stuffy nose from a cold responds to something spicy (fire) that melts and moves the mucus.

If it's dry, moisten it. This can be as simple as using a moisturizer (water) on your skin. It can also be drinking more water and ensuring you get adequate quality oils to ease chronic dryness resulting in constipation or other imbalances.

If it's wet, dry it out. Diarrhea responds to increased fiber (earth) to soak up the excess water. Edema can respond to massage (fire) to move the water.

If it's too tense, relax it. Cramps respond to massage or heat. (air and fire) Nervous tension can be calmed with deliberate breathing (air) and grounding exercises (earth).

If it's too relaxed, tighten it. Incontinence can respond to exercises to strengthen the muscles (fire and earth). Depression responds to exercise. (fire)

This framework may seem simplistic initially, but it becomes more intuitive after a while. As you read the properties of each element in your You Playbook, you begin to see how those elements show up in your constitution and your imbalances.

It's elementary, Watson!

The next piece of the puzzle is how the elements correspond to the parts of the plant. Let's start at the root and work our way up.

What element do you think corresponds with the roots of a plant? Earth! You knew that intuitively, didn't you? What are some root vegetables? Sweet potato, beets, onions, turnips, radishes, potato, malanga, cassava, etc.

Root vegetables are also high in fiber and full of prebiotics. Prebiotics feed the very important probiotics in your gut. When you think of the earth element, think of dense, building, and grounding. Earth can bank a fire or soak up excess water. It can ground air and give some solidity to ether.

Now, the stem of the plant. What does the stem do? It transports water! Stem corresponds to the water element. Think of electrolytes and how important they are in the fluids in the body. Asparagus, collards, and celery are examples of stems that nourish the water element.

Water is also found in many vine fruits. Think watermelon, cucumber, etc. The water element can cool fire, help earth become more fluid, and moisten ether and air.

The leaves of a plant correspond to the air element. Leafy greens are an easy example, and you can experience how you feel lighter after a leafy salad. Air can lessen the density of earth, dry up excess water, and create movement in ether and fire.

The flower is considered to be the fire of the plant. We don't often eat flowers in this culture but think of nasturtium, mustard, and herb flowers. Fire is an obvious element that is easy to find in our diets. Spices like red pepper, cinnamon, ginger, etc bring fire to a dish.

The last element can be found in seeds. When you gaze up at space, you see it contains everything. Planets, stars, and gal-axies are all contained in space. So, too, a seed contains all of the plant that it will become. Therefore, seeds are considered to correlate with the ether element.

Some Tasty Information

Here is the final key to your secret formula. You don't have to memorize this because your You Playbook will walk you through it. It's good to see the framework, so when you get there, it makes sense.

Let's talk about your tongue. Your food experience starts at the nose, but the real magic happens on your tongue. You have between 2,000 and 8,000 taste buds. They aren't just there for your enjoyment.

Each flavor has a different effect on the body. Salt makes you thirsty and encourages you to drink, It's also vital for many other reasons, having to do with electrolytes and water balance in your body.

Spicy makes you sweat and increases circulation. Sweet cools you down. Bitter signals your digestive system to secrete bile.

Your tongue also does something very, very important. It tells you when you've had enough. Processed food is precisely engineered to bypass this signal. That's one of the many reasons that we overeat.

When we talk about sweet taste, we aren't talking about cookies and ice cream. Beets, sweet potatoes, dates, and fruits are the kinds of sweet things we're discussing.

Here is a rundown of each flavor and its impact on the body. This is another key to your formula. If we balance the elements- fire, air, earth, ether, and water, it's really helpful to know how the flavor impacts the elements.

1. Sweet

Qualities: Cooling, moistening, building.
Effects: Nourishing, tonifying, and strengthening. The sweet taste, in moderation, can build bodily tissues, increase weight, and help with weakness. It can also calm the nervous system.

Note: Overconsumption of sweet foods, especially refined sugars, can lead to dampness, weight gain, and imbalances like diabetes. Refined sugars should be avoided altogether.

2. Bitter

QUALITIES: COOLING AND DRYING.

Effects: Detoxifying, anti-inflammatory, and fever-reducing. Bitter tastes can help clear heat from the body and counter-act dampness. It can also stimulate digestion and appetite by promoting bile secretion.

Note: Too much bitter can be depleting and may lead to dryness.

3. Salty

Qualities: Warming and moistening.

Effects: Softening to hard masses or tumors, lubricating, and purging. Salty foods can promote digestion and support the kidneys and bladder. They may also have a laxative effect in higher amounts.

Note: Excessive salt can lead to hypertension, water retention, and strain on the kidneys. Salt comes in many different types, and it can be good to use a variety of salts.

4. Sour

Qualities: Cooling and astringent (drying).

Effects: Sour can help with digestion (by increasing salivary and gastric secretions) and can be tonifying, especially to the liver. The astringent quality can reduce diarrhea and excessive sweating.

Note: Overindulgence might lead to excessive constriction or dryness in the body.

5. PUNGENT/SPICY

Qualities: Warming and drying.

Effects: Promotes circulation, stimulates digestion, dispels cold, and breaks up mucus. Pungent herbs and foods can be excellent for colds, congestion, and stagnant conditions.

Note: Excessive spicy or pungent foods can increase heat and potentially harm the yin aspects of the body.

6. ASTRINGENT (IN AYURVEDA)
QUALITIES: COOLING AND DRYING.

Effects: Reduces inflammation, constricts tissues, and absorbs water. It is commonly found in legumes and certain fruits like pomegranates and bananas. Astringent foods can be helpful in cases of excessive discharge, diarrhea, and hemorrhage.

Note: Too much astringent taste can cause constipation or blockages.

Putting it all together:

Let's just do a quick review of our framework:

- Each of us is made up of a unique blend of the five elements.
- Plant parts correspond to the elements. This gives us hints on what to eat to balance our elements.
- There are different breathing techniques, movements, and things we can take in (food, thoughts, opinions) that will influence our elements.
- Different flavors impact the elements and give us another shortcut to knowing what to eat to balance our elements.

This will become clearer in the You Playbook. I found it helpful to see how traditional medicine practices put this all together and how much sense it makes. It quickly becomes intuitive, and you have the knowledge you need at your fingertips.

Intuition is simply your mind making many connections without being consciously aware of the process. Think of it as your own AI- Acute Intelligence- at work. It's when you put information into your brain, and it comes out your gut.

What will you do now?

Now you have choices. I hope I've given you the information and the tools to choose the things that are the very best for you. It's your journey from here. Go to the You Playbook, and start learning who you **truly** are.

Chapter 14

It's All About YOU

Welcome to your You Playbook!

By the end of the playbook, you will understand what elements are primary in your base constitution and what elements might be out of balance. The first series of questions is about your base constitution.

The You Playbook is a companion journal that walks you through this journey and gives you space to record your answers and insights as you go along. If you have the You Playbook, then switch over to using it now.

If you don't have the You Playbook, get paper or a notebook to record your answers.

You want to answer these questions based on what is usual for you. For example, if you've been cold most of your life but recently feel more warm, answer based on what is usual, not what might have changed recently.

You'll total up the numbers of your answers for each element. You might want to take this test multiple times as you begin implementing your Secret Formula; you may find changes. Sometimes, our primary element isn't revealed immediately if we've been out of balance for a long time.

There will be a different test for imbalances. We will look at those later.

Who are you?

AIR ELEMENT:

1. How often do you find your mind jumping from one thought to another?
   1. Rarely (2) Occasionally (3) Sometimes (4) Often (5) Always
2. How would you describe your physical activity level?
   1. Sedentary (2) Light (3) Moderate (4) Active (5) Very Active
3. How quickly do you tend to speak?
   1. Very slowly (2) Slowly (3) At a moderate pace (4) Quickly (5) Very quickly
4. How would you describe your body frame?
   1. Large/Heavy (2) Somewhat large (3) Medium (4) Slim (5) Very slim
5. How quickly do you adapt to new situations?
   1. Very slowly (2) Slowly (3) At a moderate pace (4) Quickly (5) Very quickly
6. How often do you experience anxiety or nervousness?
   1. Rarely (2) Occasionally (3) Sometimes (4) Often (5) Always
7. How would you describe your sleeping pattern?
   1. Deep sleeper (2) Somewhat deep sleeper (3) Average sleeper (4) Light sleeper (5) Very light sleeper

EARTH ELEMENT:

1. How strong is your attachment to material possessions?
   1. Very low (2) Low (3) Moderate (4) High (5) Very high
2. How would you describe your digestive system?

1. Very weak (2) Weak (3) Average (4) Strong (5) Very strong
3. How stable do you consider your emotions to be?
   1. Very unstable (2) Unstable (3) Neutral (4) Stable (5) Very stable
4. How would you describe your pace in daily activities?
   1. Very fast (2) Fast (3) Moderate (4) Slow (5) Very slow
5. How connected do you feel to nature and the environment?
   1. Not at all (2) Slightly (3) Moderately (4) Quite a bit (5) Extremely
6. How easy is it for you to gain weight?
   1. Very hard (2) Hard (3) Neutral (4) Easy (5) Very easy
7. How would you describe your skin type?
   1. Very dry (2) Dry (3) Normal (4) Oily (5) Very oily

Ether Element:

1. How imaginative or creative would you say you are?
   1. Not at all (2) A little (3) Somewhat (4) Quite (5) Extremely
2. How frequently do you meditate or engage in deep reflection?
   1. Never (2) Rarely (3) Sometimes (4) Often (5) Daily
3. How would you describe your connection to spirituality or the metaphysical?
   1. Non-existent (2) Slight (3) Moderate (4) Strong (5) Very strong
4. How often do you experience feelings of detachment or spaceiness?
   1. Never (2) Rarely (3) Sometimes (4) Often (5) Always
5. How easy is it for you to forgive others?
   1. Very difficult (2) Difficult (3) Neutral (4) Easy (5) Very easy

6. How receptive are you to new ideas and perspectives?
   1. Not at all (2) Slightly (3) Moderately (4) Quite (5) Extremely
7. How often do you find yourself daydreaming?
   1. Never (2) Rarely (3) Sometimes (4) Often (5) Always

WATER ELEMENT:
   1. How would you describe your emotional sensitivity?
      1. Very low (2) Low (3) Moderate (4) High (5) Very high
   2. How good are you at going with the flow in unexpected situations?
      1. Very poor (2) Poor (3) Average (4) Good (5) Excellent
   3. How would you describe your fluid intake daily?
      1. Very insufficient (2) Insufficient (3) Adequate (4) More than enough (5) Excessive
   4. How connected do you feel to your emotions and intuition?
      1. Not at all (2) Slightly (3) Moderately (4) Quite a bit (5) Extremely
   5. How would you describe your ability to relate to others emotionally?
      1. Very poor (2) Poor (3) Average (4) Good (5) Excellent
   6. How often do you cry or feel moved to tears?
      1. Never (2) Rarely (3) Sometimes (4) Often (5) Very frequently
   7. How would you describe your dreams?
      1. Non-existent (2) Sparse and plain (3) Moderate (4) Vivid (5) Waking dreams

FIRE ELEMENT:
   1. How would you describe your metabolism rate?
      1. Very slow (2) Slow (3) Moderate (4) Fast (5) Very fast
   2. How often do you find yourself taking initiative and leadership in group settings?

1. Never (2) Rarely (3) Sometimes (4) Often (5) Always
3. How would you describe your approach to completing tasks and goals?
   1. Laid-back (2) Somewhat relaxed (3) Moderate (4) Proactive (5) Very proactive
4. How would you describe your digestive system?
   1. Weak (2) Somewhat weak (3) Moderate (4) Strong (5) Very strong
5. How often do you find yourself feeling warm or preferring cooler environments?
   1. Never (2) Rarely (3) Sometimes (4) Often (5) Always
6. How would you rate your passion and enthusiasm in your daily activities?
   1. Very low (2) Low (3) Moderate (4) High (5) Very high
7. How often do you find yourself taking risks or seeking new adventures?
   1. Never (2) Rarely (3) Sometimes (4) Often (5) Always

Totals:
Air _____
Earth_____
Ether_____
Water_____
Fire_____

The element(s) with the highest numbers will be primary for you. It is not unusual for a person to have two equally primary elements. If you have the stand-alone You Playbook, fill in the first part of the I AM section.

Be sure not to get caught up in describing an element as good or bad. Like everything in life, every element has two sides to the coin. We are learning about the properties and using them to adjust ourselves to be the most balanced and highest expression of ourselves.

When trying to understand an element, it is good to think about how it is expressed in nature. Water is important for all of life, but too much water in the wrong place can be catastrophic.

A campfire and a forest fire are very different things. A warm summer breeze is nothing like a tornado. You get the picture. Keeping the elements within us in balance helps keep our body in homeostasis. Homeostasis is just a fancy word for balance. Every element is both good and bad.

Imbalances can be too much or too little, but in this format, we will assume that there is too much of an element. Correcting too much fire, for example, will also correct too little earth and/or water,

Now that you know, you know!

What follows in the next chapter is a description of each element. Read it through a few times, and then ask yourself these questions:

Where does this element show up most strongly in me? Does it reflect in my personality? How are my emotions driven by this element? How does this affect my thinking?

Spend some time on this. It's a self-exploration tool that can yield beautiful results.

Chapter 15

It's elementary

AIR ELEMENT
1. General Overview:

  · Air represents movement, change, and lightness. It embodies the qualities of flexibility, communication, and intellect. It's associated with thoughts, ideas, and the breath.

2. Strengths and Benefits:

  · Adaptability: Those with a strong air element can easily adjust to different situations and changes.
  · Communication: Air enhances the ability to express oneself and to connect with others.
  · Creativity and Ideas: A heightened sense of imagination and a rich realm of ideas often dominate the mind.

3. Challenges and Growth Opportunities:

  · Grounding: Air individuals might struggle to feel grounded or focused, often "in their heads."

· Consistency: Maintaining consistency can be challenging due to its changeable nature.
· Growth Opportunity: Developing mindfulness practices or grounding exercises can help anchor their energy and cultivate stability.

EARTH ELEMENT
 1. General Overview:

· Earth represents stability, groundedness, and nourishment. It's associated with the physical body, nature, and the sense of touch.

 2. Strengths and Benefits:

· Stability: Those dominated by the earth element tend to be reliable and consistent.
· Practicality: They possess a grounded approach to life and make decisions based on realism.
· Nurturing: Earth individuals often have a strong nurturing instinct, providing care and stability to those around them.

 3. Challenges and Growth Opportunities:

· Resistance to Change: They may struggle with change or anything that disrupts their stability.
· Tendency to be Overly Cautious: Might miss opportunities due to overemphasizing safety or security.
· Growth Opportunity: Embracing change and cultivating flexibility can bring a renewed sense of freedom and growth.

ETHER ELEMENT
  1. General Overview:

- Ether, also called "Space," represents the vastness, the emptiness, and the spiritual realm. It's the bridge between the physical and the non-physical.

  2. Strengths and Benefits:

- Intuition and Insight: Ether-dominated individuals often possess deep intuition and spiritual insights.
- Open-mindedness: They are typically open to new ideas and are receptive listeners.
- Connection to the Spiritual: Often have a heightened sense of spirituality or connection to higher realms.

  3. Challenges and Growth Opportunities:

- Grounding: May struggle to stay connected with the tangible, getting lost in thought or daydreams.
- Detachment: They might feel distant or detached from the world around them.
- Growth Opportunity: Engaging with the physical realm, like through tactile activities, can enhance their connection to the world.

WATER ELEMENT
  1. General Overview:

- Water represents fluidity, emotions, and intuition. It's associated with the heart, feelings, and the ability to connect emotionally.

  2. Strengths and Benefits:

- Empathy: Water individuals are often profoundly empathic and understanding.
- Emotional Depth: They can navigate the depths of emotions, both theirs and others.
- Receptivity: They are typically open and receptive, allowing them to connect deeply with others.

3. Challenges and Growth Opportunities:

- Overwhelm: They can easily become overwhelmed by their own or others' emotions.
- Boundary Issues: Might struggle to set boundaries, absorbing others' feelings.
- Growth Opportunity: Learning emotional regulation and setting clear boundaries can ensure they don't deplete their energy.

FIRE ELEMENT
1. General Overview:

- Fire represents transformation, passion, and dynamism. It's associated with energy, drive, and the will.

2. Strengths and Benefits:

- Passion: Those with a strong fire element are often deeply passionate and enthusiastic.
- Transformation: They possess the power to transform and renew situations.
- Leadership: Naturally assertive, they often take leadership roles and inspire others.

3. Challenges and Growth Opportunities:

- Impulsivity: Might act without thinking or let their passions override reason.
- Burnout: Their intense energy can lead to burnout if not channeled properly.
- Growth Opportunity: Cultivating patience and reflection can help harness their energy in a balanced way.

Now, let's look for any imbalances. You'll do the same thing with these questions, but now we are looking to understand things that are happening more recently but haven't been part of the way you usually are.

Many things can change the way the elements show up. Imbalances can reflect external changes that require us to make adjustments.

Here is the questionnaire for your imbalances:

Air Element:

1. How often do you experience dry skin or dry eyes?
   1. Never (2) Rarely (3) Sometimes (4) Often (5) Always
2. How frequently do you find yourself lost in thoughts, unable to focus on the present moment?
   1. Never (2) Rarely (3) Sometimes (4) Often (5) Always
3. How often do you struggle with insomnia or restless sleep?
   1. Never (2) Rarely (3) Sometimes (4) Often (5) Always
4. How prone are you to experiencing anxiety and nervousness?
   1. Never (2) Rarely (3) Sometimes (4) Often (5) Always
5. How often do you have digestive issues like bloating or gas?
   1. Never (2) Rarely (3) Sometimes (4) Often (5) Always

EARTH ELEMENT:
1. How often do you feel overly attached to or possessive towards things or people?
   1. Never (2) Rarely (3) Sometimes (4) Often (5) Always
2. How frequently do you experience sluggish digestion or constipation?
   1. Never (2) Rarely (3) Sometimes (4) Often (5) Always
3. How often do you feel stuck, unable to embrace change or new experiences?
   1. Never (2) Rarely (3) Sometimes (4) Often (5) Always
4. How often do you experience feelings of lethargy or lack of motivation?
   1. Never (2) Rarely (3) Sometimes (4) Often (5) Always
5. How frequently do you find yourself overeating or craving salty and sweet foods?
   1. Never (2) Rarely (3) Sometimes (4) Often (5) Always

ETHER ELEMENT:
1. How often do you feel disconnected or spaced out, losing touch with reality?
   1. Never (2) Rarely (3) Sometimes (4) Often (5) Always
2. How often do you experience difficulties in communicating your thoughts clearly to others?
   1. Never (2) Rarely (3) Sometimes (4) Often (5) Always
3. How frequently do you struggle with feeling grounded and stable in your daily life?
   1. Never (2) Rarely (3) Sometimes (4) Often (5) Always
4. How often do you feel uninterested or apathetic towards physical activities or the material world?
   1. Never (2) Rarely (3) Sometimes (4) Often (5) Always
5. How frequently do you experience feelings of loneliness or isolation?
   1. Never (2) Rarely (3) Sometimes (4) Often (5) Always

WATER ELEMENT:

1. How often do you feel emotionally overwhelmed, as if you carry too much emotional weight?
   1. Never (2) Rarely (3) Sometimes (4) Often (5) Always
2. How frequently do you experience fluid-related issues such as water retention or urinary problems?
   1. Never (2) Rarely (3) Sometimes (4) Often (5) Always
3. How often do you find it difficult to set boundaries and say no when necessary?
   1. Never (2) Rarely (3) Sometimes (4) Often (5) Always
4. How frequently do you experience cold hands and feet or a general feeling of being cold?
   1. Never (2) Rarely (3) Sometimes (4) Often (5) Always
5. How often do you struggle with feelings of insecurity or fear?
   1. Never (2) Rarely (3) Sometimes (4) Often (5) Always

FIRE ELEMENT:

1. How frequently do you experience inflammatory issues such as redness, heat, or swelling in the body?
   1. Never (2) Rarely (3) Sometimes (4) Often (5) Always
2. How often do you find yourself experiencing bouts of anger or irritability?
   1. Never (2) Rarely (3) Sometimes (4) Often (5) Always
3. How frequently do you struggle with impulsive behavior or making rash decisions?
   1. Never (2) Rarely (3) Sometimes (4) Often (5) Always
4. How often do you experience heartburn, acid reflux, or other fiery digestive issues?
   1. Never (2) Rarely (3) Sometimes (4) Often (5) Always
5. How often do you struggle with feelings of jealousy or envy?
   1. Never (2) Rarely (3) Sometimes (4) Often (5) Always

We'll use the same scoring system:

Totals:

Air _____

Earth_____

Ether_____

Water_____

Fire_____

The higher numbers will point to your imbalances. When we begin our vibrant wellness journey, it is very common to have many or all of the elements out of balance. You want to work with the highest scores first.

Put those results in your I AM section under week two in your You Playbook or on a separate piece of paper if you don't have the Playbook.

If your primary element is also one of your imbalanced ones, and there is no clear leader in your other elemental imbalances, work with your primary first.

Many times, you can work on two imbalances at once. Too much fire and too little water can be the same imbalance. Add water, and the fire gets reduced.

Earth imbalances almost always affect digestion. Root vegetables are full of prebiotics and fiber. If constipation is a problem, prioritize that, as poor gut health can cause many other problems.

How do I balance all this?

Now, we get to the heart of the matter. Some of this will be intuitive. Remember, nobody knows your body like you do.

You'll find breathwork, movement, and intake recommendations for each imbalance in the following chapter. Remember, the YouTube channel has all of these demonstrated, so let's do it together for the first few times.

Chapter 16

Finding My Balance

Air Element

BREATHWORK

- Alternate Nostril Breathing (Nadi Shodhana): Helps balance the brain's left and right hemispheres and create a sense of calm.
- Bhramari Breath (Bee Breath): This can be soothing and helps to reduce anxiety, a common issue with air imbalance.

MOVEMENT

- Yoga poses promote grounding, such as Mountain Pose and Child's Pose.
- Slow, controlled Tai Chi movements can help in grounding the air element.

FOOD

- Root vegetables, like carrots, beets, and sweet potatoes, can promote grounding.
- Warm and cooked foods: Avoid raw and cold foods to counteract excess air element.

AFFIRMATIONS:
- "I am grounded, focused, and at peace with the world around me."
- "With each breath, I draw in stability and release uncertainty."

Earth Element

BREATHWORK
- Kapalabhati (Skull Shining Breath): Helps energize the body and counter lethargy.
- Sitali Breath (Cooling Breath): This can help bring a light and fresh perspective, mitigating the stagnant energy of excess earth.

MOVEMENT
- Backbends in yoga, like Cobra Pose or Upward Facing Dog, can introduce energy and fluidity.
- Dynamic dancing: Encourage fluid movement and break up stagnation.

FOOD
- Leafy greens, like kale and spinach, can counter heaviness.
- Spicy foods: These can help in stimulating digestion and breaking up stagnation.

Affirmations:

"I am adaptable, flowing effortlessly through changes and challenges."

- "I nurture myself with loving kindness, welcoming lightness and vitality into my body."

Ether Element

BREATHWORK

- Ujjayi Breath (Ocean Breath): This can help ground and focus the mind.
- Dirga Breath (Three-Part Breath): Helps connect with the physical body and ground excess ether.

MOVEMENT

- Stability and balancing poses, like Tree Pose or Warrior III in yoga, can help in grounding excess ether elements.
- Strength training: Focus on exercises that build muscle and connect with the physical body.

FOOD

- Protein-rich foods, like legumes and lean meats, can help in grounding.
- Root vegetables: Incorporate more grounding foods to balance excess ether.

Affirmations:

"I am connected to my physical presence and honor the space I occupy."

- "I am grounded in the here and now, embracing the tangible and the real with open arms."

Water Element

BREATHWORK

- Bhastrika (Bellows Breath): This can be energizing and helps in reducing excess water.
- Surya Bhedana (Right Nostril Breathing): Activates the fiery energy, balancing excess water.

MOVEMENT
- Twisting yoga poses, like Spinal Twist, help in reducing water retention.
- Cardiovascular exercises include jogging or cycling to stimulate heat and reduce excess water.

FOOD
- Diuretic foods like asparagus and celery can help in reducing water retention.
- Bitter foods like kale and dandelion greens can help balance excess water.

Affirmations:

- "I am fluid, releasing what no longer serves me with grace and ease."
- "I foster inner warmth and fire, balancing fluidity with purposeful action."

Fire Element

BREATHWORK
- Sheetali Breath (Cooling Breath): Helps in cooling down excess fire.
- Chandra Bhedana (Left Nostril Breathing): Activates the cooling energy, balancing excess fire.

MOVEMENT
- Yin yoga: Slow, restorative postures can help in cooling the system.
- Swimming: A cooling and gentle exercise to reduce fire.

FOOD
- Cooling foods such as cucumbers, melons, and leafy greens can help reduce fire imbalance.
- Mint or chamomile tea can have a cooling effect on the body.

Affirmations:

- "I am calm, cool, and collected, harnessing the fiery energy within me with wisdom and restraint."
- "I radiate a peaceful glow, offering warmth and light to myself and others."

Know Yourself

Everything has positives and negatives. Learning your strengths and weaknesses allows you to grow mindfully.

We tend to lean into our strengths and try to cover up our weaknesses. There is a saying that a chain is only as strong as its weakest link. We are best served by strengthening our weaknesses. This gives us balance.

I wrote this book to give us all a different way of looking at ourselves and the people around us. We could all use more true self-love and acceptance, more understanding of how to stay healthy and balanced in a world that seems to be spinning faster and faster.

If you were standing before me, I would tell you to love yourself. I would remind you that you came here with gifts, talents, and a purpose. I would ask you to treat yourself with as much care, nurturing, and patience as you treat your most beloved.

Vibrant health is possible at any age. No matter how far down the road of chronic illness, you can improve by choosing differently. You can feel better and have more energy and love of life.

As you take this journey, there will be times when the changes are challenging. Remember Future You, and know that you have what it takes to make Future You come true, One day, you will wake up and realize that Future You is here and only gets better.

Other things to consider:

Another B:
Balance. It's what we all strive for. Work-life balance. A balanced diet. These terms get thrown around a lot. But what do they really mean for you and your best life? For someone living their passion and finding great fulfillment in how they make a living, work-life balance might happen automatically. To someone working a job they hate, it might be impossible to find.

First, it's essential to recognize that balance is never static. If you watch someone on a tight wire, the micro-movements keep them from falling. There are some outstanding lessons in that.

Balance is in every part of our lives. Having a good balance in our bodies is vital for healthy aging. Falling is a common way that older people break bones, leading to rapid decline. Using the tools in this book can completely change how you age, and your ability to maintain balance in all parts of your life will become easier.

Another M:
Meditation and mindfulness are essential practices. Finding a way to quiet the mind and go into silence is beneficial in many ways. Mindfulness is about putting your entire focus into the task at hand.

If you are cutting carrots, focus entirely on the carrots. Smell the aroma they release as you cut them. Feel the knife in your hand. Notice how the handle feels and how much pressure it takes to cut the carrot.

Life moves fast. Taking time to fully engage in your life through meditation and mindfulness can bring life back into focus.

Another I:

When I share what I've learned about wellness and herbalism, I tell people that I will put a lot of information in your head, and it will come out through your gut. Intuition is a superpower that we all have. Some of us have forgotten how to use it.

You are collecting data all the time. Some of it is conscious, and some of it is not. We have a "feeling" about something. An interaction with a person doesn't "feel" right. This isn't something supernatural or woo-woo.

It's your subconscious mind at work, sending you messages derived from data that you might not be aware of at the moment. Don't discount that data. Cultivate your intuition and lean into those feelings.

Enjoy the journey!!

-

Chapter 17

Extras

This chapter is a mishmash of things that I thought you might be interested in, but that might have bogged the book down a bit. So if you still want more. dive in:

What follows is a slight veer off the current path, but very important!

If you aren't toxin aware, EWG.org is a great place to see what's in your personal and home products. When you land on the home page, scroll down to consumer guides, and you'll find great data that can help you minimize toxin exposure.

I can control what I put in my body to help mitigate any adverse effects of toxin exposure. I have limited control over other toxins.

Many of the common toxins that we are exposed to are endocrine disrupters. These can cause you to experience weight gain, hormonal imbalances, and more. When you're experiencing health issues that don't make sense in any other context, finding ways to reduce toxicity in your life is critical.

The state of our food system in the U.S. is deplorable. Access to high-quality, deeply nutritious food is extremely limited for the average person. Understanding this is vital.

Removing toxins from your body and environment may take a while, but it's worth it. I can't even walk down the conventional cleaner aisle. My sinuses start to burn when I get anywhere near there.

I left a dentist I had been with for quite a while when they started using Glade in the waiting room. I have walked out of places where I went to spend money because of their use of toxins.

It shocks me when I see healthcare facilities using these toxic products. I have a dear, dear friend, and we sit on the patio when I visit because she uses Febreze-like products in her home, and it makes my sinuses burn. Once you get away from these chemicals, you'll quickly understand.

I look at it like this: I can only control the type and amount of toxins I am exposed to to a certain degree. Too many people are still unaware of the poisons being sold to them daily. Scented products are the worst, but toxins are hiding everywhere.

The whole system works for us.

The natural world does more for us than provide sustenance. It also feeds our souls and soothes our nervous systems.

Interacting with nature can have a wide range of positive impacts on humans. Here are some ways nature can influence us:

Mental Health Benefits: Spending time in nature has been shown to reduce stress, anxiety, and depression. The calming and peaceful environment of natural settings can promote relaxation and help alleviate mental fatigue.

Physical Health Benefits: Engaging in outdoor activities can lead to increased physical activity, improved cardiovascular health, and better overall fitness. People who regularly interact with nature are often more active, contributing to a healthier lifestyle.

Emotional Well-being: Nature can evoke positive emotions and a sense of awe and wonder. Being in natural surroundings can lead to happiness, contentment, and a deeper connection with the world around us.

Enhanced Creativity and Cognitive Function: Nature can stimulate creativity and problem-solving skills. Taking a break in natural environments can improve focus and attention, enhancing cognitive abilities.

Reduced Social Isolation: Engaging in outdoor activities can be a social experience, whether hiking with friends, joining community gardening projects, or participating in nature-based group activities. This can help reduce social isolation and foster a sense of belonging.

Improved Immune Function: Some studies suggest that spending time in nature can boost the immune system, improving the ability to fight illnesses.

Stress Reduction: Exposure to nature has been associated with lower levels of the stress hormone cortisol, indicating a reduced stress response.

Better Sleep: Spending time in natural environments and exposure to natural light during the day can help regulate the body's internal clock, improving sleep quality.

Environmental Awareness and Stewardship: Interacting with nature can cultivate a sense of appreciation for the environment and foster a desire to protect and conserve it for future generations.

Mindfulness and Presence: Being in nature often encourages mindfulness and living in the present moment. This can lead to greater self-awareness and a deeper connection with the world.

I'm about to geek out a little more on plants and what they do for us. You can skip this if you want. Your You Playbook will recommend foods that are good for you, but you'll still want to consume the widest variety of whole foods.

If you aren't as passionate about plants as I am, you can skip this part too.

Plant chemical compounds play a significant role in maintaining human health. These compounds, including polyphenols, tannins, saponins, alkaloids, and others, are bioactive substances in various plant-based foods, herbs, and medicinal plants. They contribute to plants' taste, color, and aroma and offer a wide range of health benefits when consumed by humans. Here's some more info on these wonderful phytos and some of the major classifications:

Polyphenols: Polyphenols are a diverse group of compounds found in fruits, vegetables, whole grains, tea, and cocoa. They act as powerful antioxidants, which help protect the body against damage caused by free radicals, reducing the risk of chronic diseases such as heart disease, cancer, and neurodegenerative disorders. Polyphenols also have anti-inflammatory properties, support healthy digestion, and may contribute to improved cardiovascular health.

Tannins: Tannins are a type of polyphenol found in many plant foods, including tea, coffee, wine, berries, and legumes. They possess antimicrobial properties that can help protect against certain types of bacteria and fungi. Tannins also have astringent properties, which can help alleviate diarrhea and promote wound healing. Furthermore, they have been associated with potential anti-inflammatory effects and the prevention of certain types of cancers.

Saponins: Saponins are natural detergents in various legumes, such as chickpeas, lentils, and soybeans. They have been shown to exhibit anti-inflammatory, antioxidant, and immune-modulating properties. Saponins may help lower cholesterol levels, enhance immune function, and reduce the risk of certain cancers. Additionally, they have been studied for their potential in preventing or managing obesity and type 2 diabetes.

Alkaloids: Alkaloids are a large group of nitrogen-containing compounds found in numerous plants, including coffee, tea, cocoa, and medicinal herbs such as opium poppy and cinchona bark. Alkaloids can have diverse effects on the human body, such as analgesic (pain-relieving), stimulant, or sedative properties. For example, caffeine, a well-known alkaloid, acts as a stimulant to the central nervous system, increasing alertness and reducing fatigue.

Numerous other plant chemical compounds contribute to human health. For instance, carotenoids, responsible for the vibrant colors in fruits and vegetables, are potent antioxidants and may support eye health and reduce the risk of certain cancers. Flavonoids, another group of polyphenols, have anti-inflammatory and antioxidant properties, potentially benefiting cardiovascular health and brain function.

Plant chemical compounds, including polyphenols, tannins, saponins, alkaloids, and others, are vital in maintaining human health. These bioactive compounds provide antioxidant, anti-inflammatory, antimicrobial, and other beneficial effects. Including various plant-based foods in the diet ensures an intake of these compounds and supports overall health and well-being.

I eat a largely vegetarian diet with an occasional bit of fish. I do this because that is what serves my unique constitution. It's part of my Secret Formula.

We all know that processed foods are bad for you. I won't bore you with more data on that. But I will suggest that you get an app like Yuka or JollyGut to give you an easy way to at

142 ~ CYNTHIA SCHAEFER

least avoid the worst of processed foods. We'll all eat something that isn't the best for us occasionally. Using those apps will keep you from putting awful things in your body

How many times have we heard: "Eat right and exercise"? Eating right in today's world requires understanding, creativity, and an ability to source healthy food. There are some substantial obstacles to that.

The first obstacle is economic. Let's look at the cost differential between whole and processed foods:

The cost of quality whole foods is about 50% more than processed foods on a strictly economic basis. There is a lot you can do about that.

Many of us are stressed by the idea of meal prep. It requires a bit of time and a bit of creativity. Like any routine, it takes a bit to get into the flow. Once we do, though, I think there are many ways to keep costs down and vastly increase the quality of the food you eat.

When it comes to food, I've found that most people find it easier to add something than to try to approach things from the idea of deprivation. One of the easiest things you can do is add a salad to your day.

When I was growing up, "salad" meant a little iceberg lettuce, a slice of tomato, cucumber, and maybe some carrot shreds. This was usually smothered in some creamy dressing.

Today, my salads are very different. Whatever is in season always goes into my salad, along with a bunch of other things. Right now, avocados are in season, along with a lot of herbs and weeds. I throw these all together with some nuts, cooked beans, berries, or whatever else strikes my fancy.

Whole foods and Whole Foods:

Why are organic whole foods so expensive? Why is Whole Foods grocery store also known as Whole Paycheck?

There are a lot of answers to those questions, but the big answer is the subsidies in the Farm Bill and what the government chooses to support. That's a rabbit hole of special interests, campaign finance, and lobbying that we all probably know about but feel helpless to change.

Interacting with the political system in this country can be frustrating. Despite almost 30% of voters being registered independents, this country has far too much single-issue and party-line voting. We know this but haven't found a way past it yet. I am confident that once enough of us understand how we can change this, it will change, but that's not what this book is about.

We could write a book on subsidies, special interests, and how big corporations lobby to get soda approved for snap programs, but let's keep this simple.

Corn subsidies result in some form of corn being found in most processed foods. In the form that is usually used in processed food (high fructose corn syrup), it brings no value except caloric, and the downside of the insulin spike that results is driving a lot of the chronic diseases in our country,

Historically, corn has been one of the most heavily subsidized crops in the United States.

In recent years, the U.S. government has spent billions of dollars annually on corn subsidies. For example, in fiscal year 2020, the U.S. Department of Agriculture (USDA) provided approximately $5.5 billion in direct payments and other support to corn farmers. It's important to note that this figure represents the total support provided to corn farmers and includes various programs such as price support, crop insurance, and conservation programs.

It's worth mentioning that the specific amount allocated to corn subsidies can vary over time due to changes in government policies, shifts in agricultural priorities, and evolving economic conditions.

We have to include food quality in our equations. Simple calories to keep people alive are vitally important, but if those calories drive chronic illnesses and bankrupt our future, we must rethink it.

If capital and will were put behind the problem, we could quickly solve it.

One of the keys to food quality also reverberates strongly on human-driven climate change. Regenerative agriculture is the new term that means farming the way it's been done for thousands of years. This is how we should be farming. Instead, we use industrialized methods and monocrop. More on that:

Here's why the current industrialized monocropping system is problematic: Monocropping, which refers to the practice of growing a single crop on a large scale, and conventional food growing methods have several problems that impact the quality of the food and have negative consequences for both human health and the environment.

Nutrient Depletion: Monocropping can lead to nutrient depletion in the soil. When the same crop is grown continuously without rotation or diversification, it depletes specific nutrients from the ground, resulting in diminished nutrient content in the harvested crops. As a result, the quality and nutritional value of the food produced may be compromised, leading to potential nutrient deficiencies in the human diet.

Pesticide and Chemical Use: Conventional food-growing methods rely heavily on synthetic pesticides, herbicides, and fertilizers to control pests and weeds and promote crop growth. The use of these chemicals can have harmful effects on human health. Prolonged exposure to pesticides has been associated with various health issues, including increased risk of certain cancers, hormonal disruptions, neurotoxicity, and adverse effects on the immune and reproductive systems.

Reduced Biodiversity: Monocropping contributes to a loss of biodiversity. Large-scale monoculture systems often require clearing natural habitats, leading to the destruction of eco-systems and the loss of plant and animal species. This bio-diversity loss disrupts the ecological balance and reduces the availability of diverse food sources, including traditional and indigenous crops essential for maintaining dietary diversity and resilience.

Soil Erosion and Degradation: Monocropping can lead to soil erosion and degradation. Continuous cultivation of the same crop on a large scale can deplete soil nutrients, reduce soil organic matter, and degrade soil structure. This makes the soil more prone to erosion by wind and water, leading to the loss of topsoil, decreased soil fertility, and reduced capacity to retain moisture. Soil erosion affects crop productivity and contributes to environmental problems such as sedimentation in water bodies and reduced water quality.

Water Pollution and Depletion: Conventional agriculture practices, including monocropping, often involve using irriga-tion systems and chemical inputs that can contribute to water pollution and depletion. Excessive use of fertilizers and pesti-cides can leach into water bodies, contaminating water sources and harming aquatic ecosystems. Moreover, monocropping's high demand for water can exacerbate water scarcity, espe-cially in regions with limited water resources.

Climate Change Impact: The intensive use of synthetic fertilizers, fossil fuel-based machinery, and land-use changes associated with monocropping and conventional agriculture contribute to greenhouse gas emissions and climate change. Additionally, the loss of biodiversity and degradation of soils associated with these practices reduce the capacity of eco-systems to sequester carbon, further exacerbating climate change.

To address these problems, alternative farming practices such as organic farming, agroecology, and regenerative agri-culture have gained attention. These approaches promote

biodiversity, soil health, and reduced chemical inputs, resulting in higher-quality food, improved soil fertility, and reduced
environmental impacts. Organic farming, in particular, pro-
hibits synthetic pesticides and fertilizers, focusing on natural
and sustainable methods to maintain soil health and produce
nutritious food.

Transitioning to more sustainable and diversified farming
systems, supporting local and organic food production, and
promoting sustainable agricultural practices can help mitigate
the negative impacts of monocropping and conventional food
growing. Such changes can lead to improved food quality, reduced chemical exposure, enhanced biodiversity, and greater
resilience in climate change while promoting human health
and a healthier planet.

Regenerative agriculture is an approach to farming that emphasizes the holistic regeneration of ecosystems, soil health,
and biodiversity while promoting sustainable food production.
It goes beyond sustainable practices by actively restoring and
revitalizing degraded land, improving soil fertility, and enhancing ecosystem services. Regenerative agriculture not only has
positive environmental impacts but also has the potential to
improve the nutritional quality of the food produced.

*Here are critical aspects of regenerative agriculture and its
impact on nutrition and the environment:*

Soil Health and Nutrient Density: Regenerative agriculture
prioritizes building healthy, fertile soils through cover cropping, crop rotation, composting, and minimal tillage. These
practices promote the increase of organic matter, beneficial
soil microorganisms, and nutrient cycling. As a result, regeneratively grown crops are often richer in essential nutrients,
including vitamins, minerals, and antioxidants, compared to
conventionally grown counterparts. Improved soil health leads
to enhanced nutrient availability, which can positively impact
the nutritional quality of the food harvested.

Biodiversity and Ecological Resilience: Regenerative agriculture promotes biodiversity by integrating diverse crops, agroforestry systems, and natural habitats within farming landscapes. This approach provides beneficial insects, birds, and other wildlife habitat, creating a more balanced and resilient ecosystem. Biodiversity supports natural pest control, reduces the need for chemical inputs, and enhances pollination services, leading to healthier plants and improved crop yields.

Water Management and Conservation: Regenerative agriculture emphasizes water conservation and efficient use. Practices such as contour plowing, water harvesting, and cover crops help retain moisture in the soil, reduce water runoff, and enhance water infiltration. By promoting soil health and water retention capacity, regenerative agriculture mitigates drought impacts, improves water quality, and reduces the need for excessive irrigation.

Carbon Sequestration and Climate Change Mitigation: One of the significant advantages of regenerative agriculture is its ability to sequester carbon dioxide from the atmosphere and mitigate climate change. Healthy soils with higher organic matter levels can store more carbon, reducing greenhouse gas emissions. Regenerative practices such as agroforestry, rotational grazing, and cover cropping enhance carbon sequestration, contributing to climate change mitigation.

Reduced Chemical Inputs and Pesticide Use: Regenerative agriculture minimizes or eliminates synthetic chemical inputs, including pesticides and fertilizers. Instead, it emphasizes natural and organic methods for pest control, nutrient management, and soil fertility. By reducing the reliance on chemical inputs, regenerative farming minimizes the risks of chemical residues in food and protects the environment from pollution and the negative impacts of synthetic chemicals.

Enhanced Resilience and Sustainability: The regenerative approach promotes farming systems more resilient to climate variability, pests, and diseases. By diversifying crops, incorporating agroforestry, and building healthy soils, regenerative agriculture can better withstand extreme weather events and adapt to changing environmental conditions. This resilience contributes to long-term sustainability, ensuring continued food production while minimizing negative environmental impacts.

Regenerative agriculture offers a promising pathway for sustainable food production, environmental stewardship, and improved food quality. Farmers can restore degraded lands, promote biodiversity, enhance soil health, and sequester carbon by adopting regenerative practices. In turn, these practices can lead to more nutrient-dense food, reduced chemical exposure, improved water management, and greater resilience in the face of climate change. Transitioning towards regenerative agriculture has the potential to create a more sustainable and nourishing food system for both present and future generations.

Changing over to regenerative farming can have a profound healing effect on our planet, our populations, and our futures. It is happening but probably needs to be faster to mitigate disruptions in our food supply that are likely to occur due to climate change.

To respond to climate change, we need more food growing in many places and resilient food systems to help with transitions.

What you choose matters!

AFTERWORD

I wrote this book with the help of AI. Specifically, ChatGpt and Grammerly. I know that the use of AI is controversial, and I'd like to address that. The things that have helped me and my wellness clients are principles and techniques derived from many ancient and traditional wisdom practices.

I've distilled this framework into a comprehensive but easy-to-understand system because it has been so transformational in my life and in the lives of my wellness clients and students.

I'm deeply passionate about helping people find their own peak wellness and sharing the information that will get them there.

ChatGpt was useful to help me provide the background information on how this framework evolved and to get some of the techniques outlined. This is widely known, general information and, to the best of my knowledge, is unique content generated by ChatGpt based on the wording of my questions/instructions.

As AI becomes more endemic in our lives, there will likely be better guidelines and guardrails. For me, it is a tool, and, like any tool, it can be used for good or bad. I hope you agree that my use of it was for the greater good.

Cynthia Schaefer has embodied the spirit of sustainable living, from turning her Davie, Florida, residence into an edible landscape masterpiece to founding The Caring Community, a nonprofit supporting educators and growing fresh food for local food banks.

https://thecaringcommunity.love/

Living in a solar-powered haven, accompanied by bees, chickens, and a diverse flora of edibles and medicinals, she is an author, speaker, wellness consultant, and beacon for those seeking a path to wellness and eco-conscious living.